Pelican Books
I Haven't Had to Go N

Dr Joseph Berke is a practising psychotherapist and family therapist. He is a Co-Founder and Co-Director of the Arbours Association in London, as well as Director of the Arbours Crisis Centre. The Arbours Association is a mental health charity which sponsors five households, including the Crisis Centre, where people in emotional distress can go for help and to live. The Arbours emphasizes personal intervention rather than physical restraint.

Dr Berke is the author of many books and articles, including *Mary Barnes: Two Accounts of a Journey Through Madness* (with Mary Barnes). He lives and works in London with his wife, the poet and critic Roberta Elzey Berke, and their two children, Joshua and Deborah.

Joseph H. Berke

I Haven't Had to
Go Mad Here

Penguin Books

Penguin Books Ltd, Harmondsworth,
Middlesex, England
Penguin Books, 625 Madison Avenue,
New York, New York 10022, U.S.A.
Penguin Books Australia Ltd, Ringwood,
Victoria, Australia
Penguin Books Canada Ltd, 2801 John Street,
Markham, Ontario, Canada L3R 1B4
Penguin Books (N.Z.) Ltd, 182–190 Wairau Road,
Auckland 10, New Zealand

First published as *Butterfly Man* by Hutchinson 1977
Published in Pelican Books 1979
Copyright © Joseph H. Berke, 1979

For permission to reproduce copyright material, we are
grateful to the following:
'As Empty as Eve', by Berton Roueché in the *New Yorker*,
© 1974 The New Yorker Magazine, Inc.;
and *The Great Physiodynamic Therapies in Psychiatry*, ed.
A. M. Sackler *et al.*, Harper & Row, Publishers, Inc.

Made and printed in Great Britain by
Richard Clay (The Chaucer Press) Ltd,
Bungay, Suffolk
Set in Linotype Times

To Dr Morton Schatzman

Contents

   Acknowledgements 9
   Preface 11
1 Madness is Not Fun 13
2 Drugs: The Girl Who Wouldn't
   Stop Singing 36
3 ECT: The Slaughterhouse Discovery 58
4 Psychosurgery: 'I Canna Hear the
   Buggas No More' 89
5 The Butterfly Man 115
6 'I Haven't Had to Go Mad Here' 133
7 The Green Hand 159
8 Families by Choice 175
9 The End of Isolation 195
   Appendices 209
   Index 213

Acknowledgements

First, I would like to acknowledge the contribution of Dr Morton Schatzman. Much of the work I describe in this book is about the Arbours Association which he founded with me in 1970. Since then his active interest and involvement in the project has helped to sustain its growth and creative development. I am further indebted to him for the references he suggested which have added to the richness of the book as well as his critical reading of all the material and his editorial advice.

I am grateful to my wife, Roberta Elzey Berke, a co-founder of the Arbours Association, with whom I discussed the manuscript at length and who was a great support to me; and to Vivien Millett, a co-founder of the Arbours Association and coordinator of its multifarious activities.

I would like to thank all the members of the Arbours network, past and present, who have contributed in many different ways to the work I have described, and especially Richard Goldberg, a co-founder, Tom Ryan, Sally Berry, Andrea Sabbadini, Laura Forti, William Saunders and Gregorio Kohon, all of whom spent considerable time discussing their work at the Arbours Crisis Centre and communities with me.

Moreover, I would like to thank all the people who discussed their experiences while resident at an Arbours community, or other community, or at hospital while struggling

I Haven't Had to Go Mad Here

with an emotional breakdown. In order to ensure their anonymity I have taken care to change their names, occupations and any other personal details as may be appropriate without detracting from the essential facts of their life experiences.

I am also indebted to my many friends and colleagues who provided material for this book, or read parts of the manuscript and gave their comments and criticisms or were otherwise helpful with their ideas and suggestions. They include: David Annesley, Mary Barnes, Dr Colin Brewer, Dr Norman Cohen, Dr Hans W. Cohn, Michael Dempsey, Dr James S. Gorden, Dr Dennis Jaffe, Dr Colin James, Elly Jansen, Dr Allen Krebs, Catherine Kuster-Ginsberg, Dr Henry L. Lennard, David McDonald, Alma Menn, Dr Loren R. Mosher, Dr Leon Redler, Dr David E. Smith, Ruthie Smith, and Dr Ross V. Speck.

I would like to thank my literary agents, Nick Emley and Stephen Davies, for all their help with the trials and tribulations of seeing this book through to publication. I am especially grateful to Charles Clark, Managing Director of the Hutchinson Publishing Group, for commissioning the book and for his encouragement and advice with every aspect of it. Also my thanks go to his assistants, Julian Watson and Jane Judd, and to the late Virginia Hilu of Harper and Row, Publishers, Inc.

Jane de Mendelssohn prepared the manuscript, and I am most appreciative of her work.

Preface

The butterfly begins as an earthbound creature which must pass through a period of physical dissolution before attaining its splendid wings and ability to fly.

The Butterfly Man, John, was initially a weak, despairing young man. Then, under pressure from within and without, he shed all trappings of normality and passed through a period of psychic fragmentation and dramatic reverie before achieving a new and vital relationship with himself and the world. During this metamorphosis he literally saw himself as a caterpillar who needed a cocoon in which to become a butterfly.

John's choice of symbols was not a coincidence. The life cycle of the butterfly has tantalized the unconscious of mankind for thousands of years. It personifies the movement from dependency to autonomy, from impotency to potency, from death to rebirth, and the wish to undergo such a transformation.

This book is about John and people like him who seem impelled to retreat from all outer concerns into an inner world of space and time removed from all usual constraints and prohibitions. It has been my repeated observation that this journey and the experiences associated with it are not inherently harmful. They can provide an opportunity for personal growth and development, as well as collapse and chaos. What happens depends, to a great extent, on the attitudes of the person who is experiencing the world in an altered manner and of those to whom he or she has turned for support. If the latter, whether professionals or not, are frightened by unusual or odd states of mind or patterns of behaviour, then they are likely to interpret them as signs of a 'mental illness' which needs to be treated, that is, stopped. On the other hand, if the person and those about him can tolerate and respect what is taking place, then a natural stage of healing and readaptation may follow.

In the first chapters I point out that the transformation of the psyche is not fun. Those who have entered the breakdown phase may do anything to have it stopped, even to the extent of yielding responsibility for their lives to complete strangers. These people, in turn, are likely to make strenuous efforts to control what they see as 'madness', first by ostracism and subsequently by hospitalization. Drugs and electric shock are further attempts at control and restraint. If these treatments do not produce the desired effect, psychosurgery may be performed. The resulting destruction of brain tissue is a direct and potentially irreversible attack on the alleged source of the disturbance, the psyche, which itself has often been represented as a butterfly.

The alternative is to allow the metamorphosis to take place. The second half of this book is concerned with the human equivalent of the butterfly's chrysalis – the sacred cave, the sanctuary, the retreat, the crisis centre or any supportive environment where a person can reconstitute himself mentally, physically and spiritually, and re-establish his life with insight different from those who had never embarked on such a voyage.

1 Madness is Not Fun

Joyce fled to the Arbours from a hospital in Chicago. She knew that her parents were arranging for her to be transferred to a sanitorium for long-term confinement, so she left the little room where two months of drugs had done her no good, borrowed some money from a friend, and caught the first available flight to London.

Joyce's grandfather was an Italian immigrant who had made a good living selling cheese. Her father, even more successful in business, was an immensely proud man who expected his children to follow in his footsteps. Long ago, he had decided that his first-born child, whether boy or girl, would become a lawyer. Joyce grew up fully aware of her anticipated career and seemed to thrive. She did well in high school and initially enjoyed university, but after her first year she found it hard to keep up; her thoughts wandered and concentration was difficult. She resented her father's all-pervasive attempts to dominate her life.

Before the start of her second-year exams, Joyce left university. Without much explanation she returned home, keeping odd hours endlessly watching television. She had little to do with either her parents or younger brother and sister. By the time Joyce had passed several months in this way, her father had exhausted both bribes and threats. Frantically, he began to drag Joyce from doctor to doctor to find out what was the matter. The diagnoses flew thick and fast, but as far as the family was concerned they were either inconsistent, inconclusive or incompatible with its collective self-image. Joyce agreed to go to a general hospital for tests. Dozens of finger pricks, X-rays and EGGS later, she was transferred to the psychiatric ward for treatment.

By chance Joyce was assigned a consultant who was open-minded and was willing to listen to her version of events. Moreover, he acceded to her request for minimal tranquillization. She met him daily and for the first time unburdened her anxieties about her family. In turn, at least one member of the family called once a day and unburdened his preoccupation about Joyce.

'She's crazy!'

'Don't believe a thing she says!'

'Everyone loves her!'

'Get her into shape soon, or else!'

While recognizing that she was very upset, the doctor did not think that a diagnosis of 'paranoia' did justice to Joyce, or explained her condition. He saw that she had an urgent need to separate from parents who were intrusive, overbearing and menacing. He discussed the issue of autonomy with her, gave her books to read on psychiatry, and suggested several places, including the Arbours Association in London, where she might find a respite from familial, if not personal pressures.

In consequence her parents fired the consultant and warned him never to speak to her again. A new doctor was called in. He prescribed high doses of tranquillizers and put the girl on strict bed rest. Of her own accord Joyce decided to leave.

When she arrived at the Arbours Crisis Centre, a retreat for people in severe distress, her speech was tremulous, her breathing heavy. Every call, every knock on the door was meant for her; any minute her parents would arrive and carry her away. My assurances did little to calm her fears: 'In England you have passed the age of consent. As you came here voluntarily, no one can take you away. No one can force you to see them, speak with them, eat with them, or be treated by them. You are perfectly safe. Look, you have been here three days and nothing has happened.'

It was the lull before the storm. On the fourth day friends of the family who 'happened' to be in London began to call the centre. All they wanted was a few words with Joyce. She locked herself in her room.

A 'business acquaintance' of the father stopped by for a chat. Joyce hid in the office. Tom and Sally, a professional couple resident at the centre, were polite but firm. Yes, they would convey the wishes of the visitors to Joyce. No, she does not want to speak to anyone now. No, she is not starving, nor in grave moral or physical danger.

Then the letters and telegrams from the parents and their lawyers began to arrive, both at the homes of people associated with the centre and at the centre itself.

'Do you realize that a sick girl is being kept from treatment?'

'Do you realize that a family is grieving?'

'Do you realize that Joyce is not responsible for her actions?'

Over the next few weeks, most of these questions were answered, perhaps not to the parents' total satisfaction, but sufficiently to alleviate their immediate concern. Yet, nothing that was said or done, no amount of discussion or personal contact, could persuade the family that Joyce knew what she was doing, that she could make her own decisions, that she could manage her own affairs. The parents were confirmed in this opinion by the many people they consulted about Joyce – relatives, friends, doctors and lawyers. All shared a similar lifestyle and outlook and could not believe that Joyce would voluntarily relinquish the possibility of becoming a rich, influential and successful lawyer. To them, anyone who seemed to make such a decision was not of sound mind, and therefore, was *sick*.

What they denied was that Joyce had never been granted responsibility for any facet of her life which impinged upon the family's values or interests. The problem was not that she had made the wrong decision, but that she had not made any decision at all. The family was furious with Joyce for breaking unspoken rules about power and authority. But her parents did not express this anger; in doing so, they would have revealed their own vulnerability to changes in the status quo. Instead they chose to undo their daughter's bid for autonomy by challenging her capacity, and her right, to make any decisions or to be responsible for herself in any way. This was to be accomplished by certifying her as mad and arranging for her to be institutionalized.

Joyce realized these designs and was desperately trying to wriggle out from under them. However, she had great difficulty in doing this because, in part, she felt constrained by the same rules as they did. She couldn't reveal her fury with them, nor could she reveal how guilty she felt about assuming a responsibility which had never been granted to her. Hence, Joyce gave up university in order to return home and mope about and later allowed herself to be infantilized by being sent to hospital; in this way she hoped to deny the responsibility she had assumed. At the same time she concealed her anger towards her parents and relatives by attributing what she felt to them. (Her experience was that they were trying to annihilate her. This represented her perception of their conscious and unconscious intentions as well as a projection of her wish to destroy them.) The result was an overwhelming sense of persecution which made it exceptionally difficult for her to confront her persecutors (the family and its agents) and avoid being invalidated by them.

The conflict continued to London. On one side were her parents who were still determined to strip her of responsibility for the running of her life. On another side was Joyce, a sad, guilt-ridden child who wished to abdicate all responsibilities for herself and be looked after by Tom, Sally or anyone else. And on the third side was Joyce, an angry, stubborn young woman who was determined to maintain her autonomy and develop her identity. The question was whether Joyce would be seen, labelled and treated as if mentally ill.

Responsibility for a person's own body, mind and actions has long been a key factor in the development of the concept of mental illness and its application. In the eighteenth century there were many doctors and others who were distressed by the exceptional punishments administered to people who manifested bizarre and socially upsetting behaviour because they were allegedly possessed by evil spirits. In order to ameliorate this physicians argued that 'madmen' should be considered as mentally infirm and not as evil. Since the physically infirm were not held responsible for what they did under the influence of their illness, the mentally infirm could hardly be held responsible for what they thought, felt or did. Instead, the 'insane' should be given care and consideration that might be extended to any sick person.[1]

Later the mantle of 'illness' was extended to people who had clearly committed criminal acts. Perhaps the most famous case was that of Daniel M'Naghten. In 1843 he shot the private secretary to Sir Robert Peel, his intended victim.

The defence was insanity. Medical evidence was introduced showing that M'Naghten was 'labouring under an insane delusion' of being hounded by enemies, among them Peel. The jury found him 'Not guilty, on the ground of insanity'.[2]

However, there was a price to pay in these and other cases where medical concepts have been used to mitigate social dilemmas. Once a person had yielded responsibility for one aspect of his life, he was certain to be stripped of responsibility for others. If the witch, subsequently declared 'mentally ill', avoided the inquisitor's rack, she did not avoid sequestration of her legal and personal rights. If M'Naghten avoided the hangman, he did not avoid involuntary residence in the Bethlehem Hospital (earlier known as 'Bedlam') for the remaining twenty-two years of his life.[3]

Today it is debatable whether the giving up of responsibility for one's thoughts, feelings or actions leads to a diagnosis of mental illness or vice versa. Certainly the one can lead to the other. A lot depends on the manner in which the transactions occur. If Joyce had confronted her parents directly with her decision, it is unlikely that she would have been immediately taken to a psychiatrist. Instead, there would have been an explosive row in the family with mutual threats, insults, recriminations and other expressions of verbal or physical abuse. Many people choose to occupy or allow others to cast them in the role of mental patient specifically to avoid such an outcome. Thereby they or their relatives are able to deny or disguise the enmity they harbour as well as the reasons for it.

The following exchange demonstrates how convenient the

concept of mental illness can be for a parent who wishes to hide hostility towards her daughter.

MOTHER: 'I don't blame you for talking that way. I know you don't really mean it.'

DAUGHTER: 'But I do mean it.'

MOTHER: 'Now dear, I know you don't, you can't help yourself.'

DAUGHTER: 'I can help myself.'

MOTHER: 'Now dear, I know you can't because you're ill. If I thought for a moment you weren't ill, I would be furious with you.[4]

Any situation involving the assumption or attribution of mental illness is an exercise in social invalidation involving two sides. One is the State, including State institutions such as the family, the school system, the medical profession, and representatives of the State such as parents, teachers, doctors. The other is the individual acting for himself.

Invalidation means both a making null and void, as of a social contract, and a making of an 'invalid', that is, a sick person. The social contract to which everyone subscribes to varying degrees is often covert. It defines the terms by which the State delegates responsibility to the individual and the terms by which the individual assumes this responsibility. A simple example occurs when a mother allows her child to walk to a near-by school by himself and the child agrees to do so. Implicit in this delegation of responsibility is the child's willingness to watch out for its own safety. If the child refuses to accept this responsibility or gives it up or if the mother decides to take it back and walk the child to school every day, then the contract will have become invalid. If the contract is not quickly resumed then the child will soon be seen as an 'invalid'. And if, over a period of time, no physical explanation is proffered and accepted by relatives, friends and neighbours, then the child will be seen as a mental invalid or as mentally ill.

There exists a pattern of giving and taking of responsibility, and giving it up and of taking it back, between the State and the individual which generates mental invalids. This pattern mirrors the exchanges which took place between Joyce and her family and provides the basis for the state of personal and interpersonal collapse which is popularly known as a 'nervous breakdown'.

An individual who suffers from a 'nervous breakdown' does not necessarily have anything wrong with his nervous system. Nor does the term reflect the degree of emotional distress that he may be experiencing. Rather it denotes a situation whereby a man, woman or child who has no obvious physical disability refuses to carry out his social and personal obligations and has to have others carry them out for him. It is a retreat from responsibility which has previously been assumed. A regression, or return to a child-like state, is an extreme form of such a breakdown.

Once a breakdown has occurred, the word 'neurotic' is often ascribed to those who, for the most part, seem to remain in touch with reality. The word 'psychotic' is often ascribed to those who, for the most part, seem to be divorced from reality. In fact, neither word provides information about the extent or the manner that a person may be in or out of touch with reality, or the realities themselves.

Significantly, there are many people who are very disturbed, whether from depression, anxiety, or other bizarre mental and physical experiences, and who are out of touch with selected areas of conventional reality but who manage to carry on with their lives. They cannot be said to have suffered or to be suffering from a nervous breakdown even though the intensity of their suffering or the degree of their perceptual deficit may be much greater than that accruing to individuals who have given up responsibility for their lives.

In contrast, some people never accept the responsibilities which others wish to give them. This rejection of responsibility leads to another form of mental invalidity which has been subsumed under the term 'behavioural disorders'. This category includes a wide variety of criminals – who are often called psychopaths or sociopaths because of their seemingly callous attacks on persons or property – perverts (according to fashion), and addicts. Once seen as or declared 'sick', these people are notoriously resistent to therapies which assume a willingness on the part of the patient to explore the reasons for his disturbing behaviour. They are far more amenable to conditioning or aversion therapy. These are treatments which are uncomfortable and may include the application of electric currents or other noxious stimuli to the body or the putting of the patient in disquieting and painful situations. In my view most of these treatments are brutal charades in which the doctor punishes people for deficient personal and social control.

Both the giving up of responsibility once assumed and the non-acceptance of responsibilities proffered are examples of the breaking of social rules. A further example of rule breaking occurs when a person tries to assume responsibilities which have not been offered. When this is done openly, there may follow a political conflict. If this is done covertly, a psychiatric conflict may ensue. The latter occurs when the State or its agents attempt to deal with the rule breaker by invalidating his actions, rather than punishing or otherwise confronting him. If the challenger acquiesces to the psychiatric invalidation, then the challenge as well as the conflict tends to be hidden. If not, then both may be brought out into

21

the open until the conflict is resolved or the challenger submits.

A frequent example of this occurs when the sexual development of an adolescent is opposed by his parents. Either the child or the parent eventually gives way, or the parents may use their authority to prevent the child's sexual expression by stripping him of responsibility for his actions and by confusing the issue. One young man I know was deemed schizophrenic by his family's doctor because, over his parents' objections, he bought Italian stiletto shoes, instead of a more conservative pair. Underlying his psychiatric invalidation was his wish to become sexually active and his parents' fervent opposition to this.

Sometimes the psychiatrist will be invoked when the State wishes to change an overt conflict into a covert one. This allows the State to deny that a challenge to its authority has taken place by declaring political and social dissenters to be mentally ill. Many Soviet dissenters have been dealt with in mental hospitals, but it is less known that this practice has also been followed in the West.[5] During the time of CND and the nuclear bomb protests in America and Europe I knew of several instances where demonstrators were sent to mental hospital instead of jail.

The prime breaker of rules is the person who has been diagnosed schizophrenic. Typically this individual will have given up responsibility for large parts of his life, not accepted it in others and taken on too much in still other areas. He will be considered mad, foolish, bizarre, unintelligible and irrational, and may become the envied emissary of his companions' darkest wishes as well as the focus of their fears. The 'schizophrenic' is a social pariah and a psychiatric wonder. Who else is the fevered beneficiary of so much speculation and the frustrating recipient of so much treatment?

Obviously the 'schizophrenic' causes considerable dis-ease in those around him. When this dis-ease is denied and thrown back on to the madman, it becomes a 'disease', a sickness called schizophrenia and confused with a psychosis. The two terms are used synonymously, but they refer to quite different phenomena.

Psychosis, as I explain in greater detail later, is an altered state of experiencing or being in reality. Schizophrenia is an expertise in producing disquiet in others, when the altered state of reality is culturally unacceptable and inadvertently upsetting. In other words, it is often against the social rules to have certain experiences or manifest certain behaviour.[6] In clinical settings these include loose associations, ambivalence, autism and inappropriate expressions of emotions.

The 'schizophrenic' may induce extreme unease in others but not have entered an altered state of reality. The converse may happen or both at the same time. In either situation the psychotic person and his schizophrenic counterpart seem to mobilize the most energetic efforts of relatives, friends and strangers to immobilize them. Such people are also masters of self-immobilization. I have chosen to emphasize their life stories in this book to illustrate the different methods of psychiatric invalidation.

Invalidation is done in two ways, by labelling and by physical restraint. Labelling includes diagnosis as well as the application of words meaning 'ill', 'foreign', 'strange' or 'no good' by one person against another. Physical restraint includes external coercion such as strait-jackets and hospitalization and internal control by means of drugs, electricity or surgery.

Labelling is most effective when performed by professionals in socially expected and accepted settings – the doctor's office, the hospital emergency room or the courtroom.

However, labelling is influential in other circumstances because it essentially consists of the magical use of words to control an anxiety-provoking person. Such a person is one who breaks social rules, primarily prevailing standards of moral and social intercourse. This leads the rule breaker to become the recipient of others' projections and the focus of their dissociated perversity and self-hatred.

Labelling is an interpersonal manoeuvre which enables a number of people, ranging from a family and its agents to a society and its agencies, to deny what they feel and to attack anyone who would arouse these denied feelings. As such it is a transpersonal defence against fear and guilt and represents the extension and transformation of an intrapsychic process, the schizoid defence of the infant, into a social event.[7] Consequently the labellers may feel free to behave towards the labelled persons – 'the chronic deteriorated schizophrenic', 'the violent psychopath', 'the social inadequate', and so on – in a cruel and destructive manner, something that could not have happened before the label had been attached.[8]

There exist enough diagnoses to cover almost the entire gamut of human experience and behaviour because there is little one can think or do that is not a potential source of anxiety to someone else. Whether a particular thought or action is subject to invalidation depends on culture, context and fashion. Currently, tens of thousands of children who are bored by school, and respond to their boredom by disrupting what they don't like, are being diagnosed as 'hyperactive', and children who run away from home are said to be suffering from a 'runaway reaction of childhood and adolescence'. Both diagnoses strip the child of responsibility for his action and deny that it might be an appropriate response to the child's social situation. Indeed, so many observers, including such distinguished anthropologists as Jules Henry, have described the destructive influence of the contemporary state school or nuclear family, that one might just as well conclude that an act of disruption or running away is a manifestation of health.[9] The children who quietly remained could then be said to be suffering from a 'passive-dependent' syndrome.

Comparably, in the nineteenth century, black slaves who tried to escape from their masters were said to be suffering from a disease called *drapetomania* and those who refused to work were considered ill with *dysaesthesia Aethiopis*.[10] In either situation a medical metaphor has been used in order to make moral, social or political judgements seem scientifically respectable.

While diagnostic metaphors may be respectable, they are not necessarily reliable. Researchers have shown that psychiatrists disagree among themselves about the diagnosis of given individuals, that psychiatrists often make different diagnoses on the same person at different times, and that the frequency of diagnosis tends to vary with different groups of patients and doctors.[11]

Diagnostic labels can also be unjust and inaccurate. In his celebrated study, Dr D. L. Rosenhan demonstrated that in a hospital setting and because of *a priori* expectations of madness, psychiatric personnel could not distinguish the sane from the insane. His experimenters gained admission to a variety of mental hospitals by falsely stating they were hearing voices. Once admitted, they stated that the symptom had gone away and they felt fine. Still, in every case, the people were diagnosed as schizophrenic and when discharged had the diagnosis 'schizophrenia in remission' appended to their charts. In a further experiment at a leading teaching hospital, Dr Rosenhan showed that the staff could not distinguish true complaints from false ones.[12]

If diagnoses are somewhat unreal, the stigmata which follow with them are not. People who have been declared or are seen as mentally ill by others become depersonalized, are ostracized from many levels of social exchange, and are bereft of many rights and responsibilities; the restrictions vary with the degree to which one has become a social nuisance. What is remarkable is that even if an individual recovers from his 'illness' – that is, plays by the social rules again, or successfully conceals that he is not playing by the rules – he may never recover all the rights and responsibilities which have been stripped from him. A new label, 'former —' which can rarely be removed remains with him. He will find that educational, employment and travel opportunities will remain closed to him.[13] Even when this person or his relatives or friends decide to forget what had previously transpired, it is impossible for them to erase his ubiquitous computer-stored case notes.

Those people who persist in disturbing others, or are seen as persistently disturbing, are subject to the application of physical restraints on their thoughts or actions. The most notable of these restraints is the deprivation of liberty by means of hospitalization. In Britain, one woman in six and one man in nine will spend some time in a mental hospital. In England, there are about 200,000 admissions per year for mental illness and the patient population in these hospitals is well over 100,000.[14]

In the United States, one in every ten Americans will spend some time in a mental hospital.[15] Each year over a quarter of a million people are committed to mental hospitals and the patient population in these hospitals is over one million.[16] Other Western countries demonstrate a comparable interests in hospitalizing large numbers of their citizens.

While labelling invalidates disquieting individuals, it provides them with a surrogate identity. Hospitalization does the same, and more. It creates an identity, the mental invalid, behind which people can hide, or be hidden; and a role, the mental patient, in which people can engage, or be forced to engage. In return, the mental patient may be relieved of responsibility for the causes of his confinement. Years ago, these causes included poverty and promiscuity. Today, they usually have to do with violence, resulting in actual or imagined damage to the patient or others.

What constitutes violence, or even damage, varies from generation to generation and culture to culture. When an act is considered to be irrational or unintelligible, then almost anything that is done may be seen as violent and damaging. When there are obvious and accepted reasons for the same act, then it may be seen as innocuous, or at least permissible. But the threat of violence or dangerousness, in general, is not the essential element in the diagnosis of mental illness or the willingness to commit someone to hospital. Rather, it is the manner or the style of the dangerousness which is important. For example, drunken drivers injure and kill many more people than persons with ideas of persecution. Yet the latter are readily sent to mental hospital, while drunken drivers are not.[17] Similarly, some forms of suicidal behaviour, like over-dosing with barbiturates, are condemned, and others, like overdosing with tobacco, are condoned.

There exists no proof that mentally or emotionally disordered individuals are more dangerous, either to themselves or others, than the population at large. On the contrary, most people wind up and remain in hospital because they are too passive, silent, fearful and withdrawn, rather than violent. This fact flies in the face of the popular notion of the 'madman' or 'maniac' who maims and kills on whim.

Many psychiatrists share this misconception, which is often based on isolated incidents blown up by the media. Consequently, they tend to overpredict danger and recommend that people be admitted to or kept in mental hospital when such restraint is not necessary.[18]

As standards of danger vary, so do the laws concerning compulsory confinement to hospital. In England, a person can be arrested and detained for seventy-two hours on the recommendation of a physician (Section 29 of the 1959 Mental Health Act) or a police officer (Section 136). He may be admitted for observation and treatment for twenty-eight days (Section 25) or one year (Section 26) with the advice and consent of two doctors.[19]

In America each state has a separate code for emergency admission to mental hospital. Some require a statement by a physician or judge attesting to mental illness and dangerousness. Others, including New York State, will allow a person to be arrested on the basis of an unconfirmed allegation by any citizen that the prospective patient is in need of treatment.[20]

In both countries there exist provisions for the non-emergency or voluntary admission of people to mental hospitals.[21] In America about ten per cent of admissions are voluntary and in England only about ten per cent are not. Yet the voluntary patient can be retained in hospital at the discretion of the attending doctor. Minimal or no provision is made for the 'informal' patient who has the absolute right to sign himself out of hospital whenever he wishes and whatever his condition.

Ironically, once a person has been admitted to hospital, the very admission becomes the strongest proof that he must be mad and deserves to be in hospital. Otherwise, as friends, neighbours and relatives ask, why would he have been admitted in the first place? This argument is generally accepted by both staff and patients as justification for the creation of a new social contract whereby the newly created patient becomes a dependent ward of an impersonal administrative bureaucracy.

This dependent relationship has been well described by Byron G. Wales, an American who spent several years as a patient in mental hospital:

It should be fairly obvious that an institution, such as a neuro-psychiatric hospital, is inherently notorious for inhibiting an individual's liberty and substituting security for freedom. Although a patient may be told that 'everything is up to you', the mere fact that medical care, food, lodging and entertainment are provided automatically impresses the patient otherwise. He is told when to rise and when to go to bed, when to eat, when to work, when to be entertained. He is given or not given ground privileges and passes to leave the confines of the hospital at the discretion of authority figures, whose power is, to all intents and purposes, absolute. And he is in most instances powerless over, and even unaware of, the criteria which influence these decisions.[22]

For his part the patient must remain docile and agree to treatment, or it will be forced. He must not question what is being done on his behalf. If he does query this, or attempts to resume personal responsibilities – such as entering a physical relationship with another patient – or asks to be released before the staff are ready to release him, then his behaviour tends to be seen as a further sign of illness, justifying continued confinement.[23]

Needless to say, the patient cannot control his space or time, his goals, his relationships, or even his own mental or physical processes (especially when given drugs or electro-shock treatment). This predicament may last for days or decades. Many patients have been locked up for thirty, forty and even fifty years.[24] Hundreds of thousands of people are currently serving indeterminate sentences in mental hospitals across America and Europe.

Prolonged hospitalization over months or years gives rise to a new phenomenon which can be described as 'institutionalism'. The patient becomes increasingly dependent on the staff for all facets of his life. His intellect dims and his facial expression becomes dull. Emotionally, he is withdrawn and apathetic, except when offered any kind of responsibility; then he becomes frightened and tremulous. This syndrome is common to individuals who have spent years in jail. Among mental patients who were admitted to hospital with a diagnosis of schizophrenia this phenomenon is know as chronic schizophrenia.[25]

Hospitalization accomplishes in a concrete manner what labelling does psychologically. The rule breaker, having been declared mentally ill and taken away to a place that is psychologically if not physically distant, is kept in confinement until his offensive activities cease, or are no longer seen to be so. Over time this person metamorphoses from someone who has committed an alien act, or demonstrated alien ideas, to an alien who used to be a person.

The deprivation of liberty is only one of a large number of civil rights which the State can withhold from 'aliens'. In England all patients, whether voluntary or involuntary, may lose the right to vote, possess a driving licence, bring civil or criminal proceedings, and many state financial benefits. They may be subject to an invasion of bodily privacy without recourse, have communications censored, and be transported anywhere in the United Kingdom without their consent. Moreover, any person who is declared to be of unsound mind may be denied the power to make a will, be a parent, or hold property. In other words, at the discretion of the Court of Protection he may be divested of virtually all control over his property and his affairs.

In the United States the loss of civil rights varies from state to state. In some, hospitalization for mental illness is synonymous with a legal decree of mental incompetence. In others a person may be declared mentally incompetent without being declared mentally ill, or vice versa. When a person is declared mentally incompetent, he can no longer enter into legal relationships with others. His signature has no value. He loses most of the basic rights of citizenship. *As a result, a mentally ill and incompetent person may have less rights than a dead man.* The latter can retain control of his property by means of his estate. The mental patient cannot even make a will. Similar restrictions exist in other countries.[26]

The deprivation of liberty, the loss of personal and civil rights, represent the institutionalized stripping of responsibility from people who have become the object of others' fear and opprobrium. It is a forcible exercise in external restraint with the collective, albeit unconscious purpose of controlling and castrating those who have broken prevailing moral, social and familial codes.

In the following three chapters I shall describe the principle methods of internal restraint: drugs, electric shock and lobotomy. All of these are further attempts at invalidating, assaulting and annihilating 'alien' thoughts and actions.

Notes

1. See discussions by Thomas Szasz, *The Manufacture of Madness* (New York, Harper & Row, 1970); Michael Foucault, *Madness and Civilization* (New York, Pantheon, 1965); and

I Haven't Had to Go Mad Here

Morton Schatzman, 'Madness and morals', *Counter Culture*, ed. Joseph Berke (London, Peter Owen, 1969), pp. 288–313.

2. Thomas Szasz, *Law, Liberty and Psychiatry: An Inquiry into the Social Uses of Mental Health Practices* (London, Routledge & Kegan Paul, 1974), p. 128.

3. The last year was spent in the Broadmoor Institute for the Criminally Insane to which he was transferred when it opened in 1864.

4. The exchange was described by Dr R. D. Laing in a discussion of mystification and quoted by Brian Inglis, 'Out of mind, out of sight', p. 63.

5. Cornelia Mee, *The Internment of Soviet Dissenters in Mental Hospitals* (pamphlet produced by the Working Group on the Internment of Dissenters in Mental Hospital, Cambridge, John Arliss, 1971). See also Roy A. Medvedev and Z. Medvedev, *A Question of Madness* (New York, Knopf, 1972).

6. See also Joseph Berke, 'Anti-psychiatry: an interview', *The Radical Therapist*, ed. J. Agel (New York, Ballantine Books, 1971), pp. 97–107.

7. For an extended discussion of the schizoid defence, see Melanie Klein, 'Notes on some schizoid mechanism', *Developments in Psycho-Analysis*, ed. E. Jones (London, Hogarth Press, 1952), pp. 292–320. Also see discussion of the transpersonal defence, Morton Schatzman, *Soul Murdered: Persecution in the Family* (New York, Random House, 1973), pp. 136–7.

8. The life of the Louisiana politician, Earl Long, provides a good example of the social rule breaker who becomes diagnosed as mentally ill and is then treated in a manner which would have been impossible before the label had been applied. In 1959 during a session of the state legislature, Governor Long broke all the taboos about mentioning sexual relations with and exploitation of blacks by white folks. He exclaimed, 'You the people that sleep with 'em at night and kick 'em in the street in the daytime.' An uproar ensued and Governor Long was subsequently railroaded into mental hospital by his wife and nephew. (Marshall Frady, 'The Longs of Louisiana', *Sunday Times Magazine*, 7 December 1975, 83.)

9. Jules Henry, *Culture Against Man* (New York, Random House, 1966).

10. Morton Schatzman, 'Psychiatry and revolution', *Arbours Network* 8 (Magazine of Arbours Association, 1975), 5–6. Schatzman quotes from the description of 'drapetomania': 'The cause, in the most of the cases, that induces the negro to run away from service, is as much a disease of the mind as any other species of mental alienation and much more curable, as a general rule. With the advantage of proper medical advice, strictly followed, this troublesome practice that many negroes have of running away, can be almost entirely prevented ...' ('Report on the diseases of physical peculiarities of the negro race', *New Orleans Medical and Surgical Journal*, 1851.)

11. See Larry Gostin, *A Human Condition* (London, National Association for Mental Health, 1975), pp. 37–8, 58–60.

12. D. L. Rosenhan, 'On being sane in insane places', *Science*, 179 (19 January 1973), p. 250.

13. In the United States it is against the law to discriminate in most jobs on the basis of a past history of mental illness. To do so is a denial of due process under the fourteenth amendment to the American Constitution. Still, this discrimination is quite frequent. See B. Ennis and L. Siegal, *The Rights of Mental Patients* (New York, Avon Books, 1973), pp. 87–8.

14. In 1973 there were about 185,000 admissions. (Sir Martin Roth, 'The age of understanding', *The Times*, 10 February 1975, p. 5.) As of 31 December 1971 there were 111,601 patients in hospital in England and Wales. (Gostin, *A Human Condition*, p. 138.)

15. Ennis and Siegal, *The Rights of Mental Patients*, p.11.

16. Szasz, *Law, Liberty and Psychiatry*, p. 40.

17. ibid., p. 46.

18. In 1966 in New York psychiatrists stated that 1,000 ex-convicts who had been diagnosed as mentally ill were too dangerous to be accommodated in ordinary mental hospitals. Subsequently, because of a U S Supreme Court decision, these people were transferred to civil (as opposed to high security) hospitals. After one year no significant problems were noted.

Many of the patients were released and the psychiatric predictions were almost uniformly wrong. (Ennis and Siegal, *The Rights of Mental Patients*, pp. 21–2.)

Other studies in England have similarly demonstrated that psychiatrists over-predict dangerousness and that many residents of high security hospitals could safely be released into the community. (Gostin, *A Human Condition*, pp. 39–42.)

19. For a full discussion of the laws concerning admission to hospital in England and Wales, see Gostin, *A Human Condition*, pp. 22–6.

20. For a full discussion and summary of the laws concerning admission to hospital in each of the fifty states, see Ennis and Siegel, *The Rights of Mental Patients*, pp. 32–9.

21. Gostin, *A Human Condition*, pp. 15–21; Ennis and Siegel, *The Rights of Mental Patients*, pp. 32–9.

22. Byron G. Wales, 'Reward of illness: observations on institutionalization by a former neuropsychiatric patient', *Mental Hygiene*, 44 (January 1960), pp. 55–63, quoted by Thomas Szasz (ed.), *The Age of Madness: The History of Involuntary Mental Hospitalization Presented in Selected Texts* (New York, Anchor, 1963), p. 268.

23. Examples of this situation are legion, ranging from people who are treated against their will to those who are wrongly detained in hospital. In England there is little the patient can do if he is not able to persuade his doctor to his point of view. Patients under a one-year order (Section 26) can apply for release to a Mental Health Tribunal. The procedure is cumbersome and unsatisfactory. See Gostin, *A Human Condition*, pp. 55–75.

In America a patient may apply for a writ of Habeas Corpus for release. Moreover, in a recent ruling the United States Supreme Court has declared that insane persons cannot be confined involuntarily if they are not dangerous and can live safely in the outside world. This decision was a personal victory for Kenneth Donaldson, a retired carpenter who was confined for fifteen years without treatment in a Florida state hospital. (*International Herald Tribune*, 28–29 June 1975, p. 5.)

24. Szasz, *Law, Liberty and Psychiatry*, pp. 198–200.

25. The equivalent of chronic schizophrenia on the staff side of the mental hospital is the backward nurse or doctor. I refer to those people who have spent years caring for chronic patients. They too are intellectually dim and rigid. Emotionally they are apathetic except when offered new responsibilities or treatment opportunities. Then they react with alarm, if not extreme cruelty, when patients or new staff do not keep to the old hospital routine. I describe one such doctor in the chapter on electroshock treatment, pp. 75–6.

26. These rights and the loss of them are discussed in great detail by Larry Gostin in the M I N D (London, National Association for Mental Health) Special Report, *A Human Condition*; Szasz, *Law, Liberty and Psychiatry*, pp. 149–90; and Ennis and Siegal, *The Rights of Mental Patients*, pp. 17–92, 93–282.

2 Drugs: The Girl Who Wouldn't Stop Singing

In New York's Greenwich Village, Karen is known and respected as a poet and singer. I first met her outside Lincoln Center, where amid a backdrop of opera house and concert hall, she intoned about love and redemption. Later I knew her as a regular at poetry readings and film shows.

One evening I heard from mutual friends that she had been picked up by the police and taken to a mental hospital. The news surprised me; Karen was eccentric, but certainly not crazy. I decided to visit her and see what was the matter.

Karen was held in the acute admission ward of a large psychiatric hospital. Visitors were unwelcome. If I had not been a physician it would have been impossible to see her. Only after a heated argument and a suspicious review of my credentials was I allowed to pass through several heavily guarded and locked steel doors. Seven floors up I entered a room bare except for a bell and another locked steel door. Muffled shouts could be heard emanating from a small barred window in the door. I rang the bell. A nurse came and opened the door, but when I told her with whom I wished to speak she recoiled in horror. 'That patient is the most dangerous person on the ward. You hear those cries? That's her. You don't want to see her!'

By now I had become apprehensive, but I pressed on down the long corridor leading to the ward. Karen was in the distance, singing, screaming and tearing at her clothes.

Then she noticed me. The wailing stopped, and she immediately ran over and gave me a big hug.

The staff was astonished. Their most difficult, unapproachable patient had changed into a friendly, affectionate human being. They offered us some coffee and a quiet corner where Karen and I could talk. She said that she had been walking along 2nd Avenue one evening on the way to a poetry reading. She had begun to sing out loud a few of the poems she was to read, when suddenly a police car came racing down the avenue and screeched to a stop right next to her. Two burly cops stepped out of the car and accosted her.

'I'm usually afraid of the fuzz. Two friends of mine have been beaten up by them for no good reason. Anyway, when those men jumped out of the car, I was terrified and just froze. Couldn't answer their questions or anything. Then they pulled me into the car and took me to the station. Then I refused to say anything. I said to myself, "Unless they apologize to me, I'm not going to tell them a thing." I don't remember much after that except waking up here and some creep forcing pills down my mouth. The pills made my mind grow fuzzy and my tongue feel big and heavy so I started to sing and shout in order to make my tongue feel better and my head clear. Then they forced me to take more pills. So I had to sing even louder. I was afraid that my thoughts would go away and I would forget who I was.'

The ward nurse confirmed that Karen had been brought to hospital by the police who complained that she was withdrawn and uncommunicative. A diagnosis of schizophrenia was made and she had been treated with Chlorpromazine (also known as Thorazine or Largactil), a strong tranquillizer, starting at 400 milligrams per day. When she started to sing and refused to sleep, the medication had been increased. Curiously, according to the nurse, this seemed to make her more frantic and by the time of my visit she was being given the massive dose of 4000 milligrams of Thorazine per day.

All the staff thought Karen's prognosis was grim. No wonder: the very treatment that they administered had the effect of making their patient frightened and socially disruptive. In turn, both doctors and nurses became frightened of Karen's real or imagined expressions of violence and of the fact that she wasn't 'getting better'. So they extended their treatment. In response, Karen became even more frightened of the effects of the drugs and redoubled her resistance to them. Consequently, both staff and patient became intensely frustrated by and frightening to the other. Each was caught in a vicious cycle of threat and counter-threat which manifested itself as pseudo-benevolence – treatment – and pseudo-illness – socially disruptive symptoms.

One simple action could have mitigated the situation. This would have consisted of a genuine attempt on the part of each side to speak to the other about its fears and difficulties. Indeed, Karen said that at the beginning of her hospitalization she tried to tell the nurses what was happening to her, but they would not listen to her. Subsequently, she decided that anything she said would be taken as a sign of her madness, so she decided not to volunteer any information.

It seems that the medical staff for its part was too preoccupied with the pressure of work and too inhibited by fear to take the trouble to ask Karen why she was singing and shouting. Yet one person did try to strike up a serious conversation with her. He was a young medical student who had just begun working on the ward. But his suggestion that Karen was not ill, just frightened by the effects and side-effects of the Thorazine, was dismissed because of his 'in-experience in such matters'.

Karen needed several weeks to recover from her treatment by the police and medical personnel. One night, while recounting her experiences on the ward, she exclaimed, 'You know something, those hospital people would have been better off taking the pills themselves. At least they might have slowed down a bit and been more willing to talk with me.'

Why are drugs in psychiatric practice at all? What do they do? Whom do they most benefit?

By psychiatric practice I mean any attempt to control and restrain the behaviour of people by 'recognized' healers, doctors, witches or priests. On many occasions there may be a thin dividing line between the work of these psychiatric authorities and that of the police authorities. For example, when morality is decided by law, rather than common consent, the role of the priest and that of the police may become interchangeable. Then the police become arbitrators of consciousness and the priest or doctor can become a purveyor of punishment.

On the other hand, most societies try to distinguish between behaviour or experience which is criminal – contrary to the continuity of the State – and that which is bothersome or frightening. Behaviour which is bothersome or frightening will not become a focus of psychiatric attention unless others are also disturbed.

A classic example is of the man who saw dinosaurs in his garden. He himself was not upset by these huge reptiles, although he did think it a bit odd that they should choose his garden in which to live. As they were herbivores, he dutifully made sure they had grass to eat and water to drink.

Otherwise he was a good husband, father and worker. One day he made the mistake of mentioning the beasts to a neighbour. The neighbour got terribly upset that anyone living next to him should be seeing dinosaurs. So he told the man's wife. The wife got terribly upset that her husband was seeing such creatures. So she called his boss. Needless to say he got upset too and they all called the doctor. The doctor did not especially care what his patients saw, but he was very annoyed by the barrage of anxious phone calls from the neighbour, wife and boss. So he insisted that the man go into hospital for treatment. In hospital the man continued to report that he saw dinosaurs and so he continued to be treated. But one day he forgot to mention the reptiles to anyone. Later he heard one of the staff telling another that he was getting better because he no longer saw his dinosaurs, though he still did. So he decided never to mention them again in the hope of getting out of hospital. This happened when he told his doctor that he no longer saw the beasts. He got his job back when the doctor reported to his boss the same. He got his wife back (from her mother) when the boss told the wife. And the neighbour came back from holiday when the wife sent him a card mentioning the new development. From then on he was careful never to tell anyone about his friends in the garden. No one was ever bothered by him again and he never had any further treatment.

The outcome of this story is highly unlikely, however. Most people who see dinosaurs are upset by what they see. Moreover, even if they were not upset by their hallucinations, they would get anxious and agitated in the face of everyone else's anxiety and agitation. Consequently, they would respond to their relatives, friends or neighbours in ways that would increase the likelihood of their being treated for something.

The moral of this story is that psychiatric problems are never a function of a single person. A 'psychiatric event' always involves a social network consisting of three sets of people : the first is the person who invokes distress in others and who may or may not be in distress himself. The second includes all the 'others' who become distressed in response to the first person's actions or lack of action and feelings or lack of feelings. (Certain people distress others, for example, by eating a lot; other people cause distress by eating very little. Alternatively, certain people cause distress by believing in God and others cause distress by not believing in God.) The third are the 'recognized' healers who choose or are chosen to reduce distress by a variety of socially acceptable treatments. These people are usually in a state of distress themselves, brought on by the original distressing person, or by the distressed 'others' or by a combination of both.

Drugs have always been one of the most popular treatments employed to reduce distress. In the old days and in different cultures folk and medicinal remedies have embraced a wide array of leaves, flowers, fruits, mushrooms and barks. Nowadays, biochemicals are used and in vast amounts. In 1967 in the United States alone, some 180,000,000 prescriptions for mind-altering drugs were written and at a cost of almost $700,000,000.[1] By 1973 these figures had risen to 214,000,000 prescriptions at a cost of over $1,000,000,000.

Invariably, these medicinal agents are given to the person who has been singled out as the cause of all the distress. The significant 'others' are never treated. Yet, if the treatment succeeds, and the distressing person changes his behaviour, it is likely that he or she will not experience the greatest relief of tension. Indeed, he may not experience any relief of tension at all, or he may even be more upset than before treatment began! Most relief will accrue to the relatives, friends, neighbours and other members of the distressing person's social circle. And as a result of their therapeutic intervention, it may be argued that the psychiatric authorities experience the greatest enhancement of well-being.

Therefore, the answer to my first question about the use of drugs is that they are used firstly to reduce tension in people who are distressed by the deeds or lack of deeds, and thoughts or lack of thoughts, of others; and secondly to enhance the well-being of those who produce, distribute and administer the drugs.

It is important to establish the way in which drugs work. Any explanations must take into account the values, expectations and beliefs common to the society in which they are employed. For example, in Europe in the Middle Ages and for hundreds of years thereafter it was common practice to prescribe emetics to induce vomiting, and cathartics to induce diarrhoea, for the mentally disturbed. By inducing vomiting and diarrhoea, people had the idea that the sick person could be induced to get rid of the evil spirits, demons, and devils which were thought to have entered body and mind and taken possession of his faculties.

These medicinals were very unpleasant, both the taste and in their physical effects. Therefore, they were used as a punitive agent. They still are. Today many mothers force their children to take laxatives when they seem irritable. One wonders whether women who do this to their children actually equate irritability with constipation or whether they secretly believe that they are driving out bad impulses from their child and punishing him to boot. Innumerable other examples could be cited in modern-day psychiatric practice. To mention one, in the treatment of alcoholism, it has been fashionable to give the patient a maintenance dose of a drug

Disulfiram which causes monumental distress – nausea, vomiting, flushing, hypertension, anxiety and palpitations – whenever he starts drinking again. It is hard to see this treatment as anything but a continual and punitive threat of internal devastation.

Also, emetics and cathartics work by exhausting a person. He becomes so tired and worn out that it is hard for him to persist with his bothersome or frightening actions. Fundamentally these drugs, as well as the wide range of tranquillizers, sedatives and hypnotics in use today, serve as a biochemical strait-jacket. This restraint expresses the wish of those who arrange for and administer these medicinal agents : total control over the disturbing person's body, mind and soul. It is also a less obtrusive but highly effective substitute for the mechanical restraints that have been utilized and continue to be utilized by the psychiatric profession.

The damage done to mental patients by external, or mechanical, restraints has been noted by many people, and in particular, the British psychiatrist, Dr John Conolly. Within four months of his appointment as resident physician of the Middlesex County Lunatic Asylum in 1839 and

without previous experience of asylum management he had abolished every form of personal restraint: 'no form of straight-waistcoat, no handcuffs, no leg-locks, nor any contrivance confining the trunk, or limbs, or any of the muscles, is now in use. The coercion chairs, about forty in number, have been altogether removed from the wards.'[2]

In 1856 Dr Conolly published *The Treatment of the Insane without Mechanical Restraints*, in which he points out that under the old system the staff saw the patient as a vicious animal that needed to be subdued. He states, 'When

43

the patient is tied up, all regard for him ceases.' And it becomes impossible to train nurses and aides to give their patients 'any show of respect, much less with any constant manifestation of humane regard'.[3]

Throughout his life Dr Conolly espoused consideration and respect for the mentally disturbed. Moreover, he continued to remain wary of most treatments, even the seemingly humane ones, for he realized there was a thin divide between treatment and restraint. His hope was that 'no future economy and no delusive theories would ever lead to the abandonment of non-restraint'.[4]

Yet, within a short time of his death, a new warning had to be sounded. This time it was by Conolly's son-in-law, the prominent psychiatrist, Dr Henry Maudsley (after whom the Maudsley Hospital in London is named). He spoke out against a new and insidious form of restraint which he called 'chemical restraint'. Maudsley pointed out that although the use of mechanical restraints had diminished, the use of sedatives in the treatment of insanity was increasing. He stated,

It is a practice which is almost universal among medical men, when they have to do with a case of mental disease, to prescribe sedatives in order to subdue excitement and to procure sleep.

He queries whether 'the putting the nerve cells of the patient's brain into chemical restraint ... did really benefit them'. He pointed out that sedatives were being used as

mechanical restraints had been unwisely used – namely to keep a turbulent patient quiet ... That is to say chemical restraint of the cells of the sick brain may be made to supersede entirely the mechanical restraint of the body. The successful argument against mechanical restraint was, that although it kept the patient's body quiet, it really aggravated his malady; the question now which should be considered is, whether chemical restraint does permanent good, or whether by diminishing excitement at the ultimate cost of mental power it makes a solitude and calls it peace.[5]

Maudsley's argument retains its validity a hundred years later. The benefits of drug therapy are ephemeral, yet the dangers remain ever present, and at a time when new and more varied forms of tranquillizers or sedatives seem to come on to the market every day, newer and more serious dangers seem to arise with each drug.

A frequent advertisement for Mellaril shows an angry lady covered by the word OBSTREPEROUS in large red letters. A claim is then made that the drug can restrain anxiety, excitement and hypermobility. In similar lettering the manufacturer notes that the drug will not repair the underlying brain damage (or, presumably, any other realistic reasons for the anger). But, significantly, most of the full-page advert is taken up by hundreds of small-type warnings, about the physical damage that the drug may cause; in other words, its side effects.[6] In the case of the Phenothiazine drugs, of which Mellaril is an example, a common and severe difficulty is muscular imbalance, discoordination or rigidity. As for what Karen experienced, the Mellaril advertisement points out that a persistent *Tardive Dyskinesia* may develop. It is 'characterized by rhythmical involuntary movements of the tongue, face, mouth or jaw and sometimes of the extremities', and may be irreversible.

A heavy price must be paid for chemical restraint. But the physical damage which may result from drug treatment represents only a more obvious part of this price. More seriously, there are the social and interpersonal costs. This includes the deliberate confusion of people who have been put in the position of patient as to the real and possibly sinister circumstances of their distress.

45

In microsocial terms we often see this happening in families where one or both parents act to diminish the autonomy of a child. In macrosocial terms it involves the elderly whose distress about money, housing, social isolation may be attributed to senile dementia rather than the miserable way that older people are actually treated in our society.

Significantly the excessive and prolonged use of psychotropic drugs may actually bring on the very syndrome for which they are being given a treatment. For example, 'flattened affect' or a bland loss of emotional response is classically considered to be a symptom of schizophrenia. Yet the Phenothiazines classically produce 'flattened affect'.

Furthermore, tranquillizers are often given to highly agitated people to calm them down. Yet, as he have seen with Karen, they may result in the opposite response where the person so treated becomes even more agitated. This can happen where a person is very frightened and continues to be frightened unless he is drugged into a stupor (then the agitation returns when the stupor wears off). The more appropriate response to agitation or violence is to help the person become aware of the fear and despair that lie behind it. When this happens, then even the most violent person will become calm very quickly.

The ability to attend to anxiety and despair presupposes the possibility of adequate communication between the distressed person and those who are trying to help him. However, drug therapy often prevents adequate communication from taking place. As Henry Maudsley pointed out, sedatives were prescribed in order to put the patient to sleep, and Chlorpromazine, the most widely used tranquillizer in the treatment of schizophrenia, was initially employed to induce artificial hibernation to facilitate anaesthesia during surgery. In fact, the two French researchers who pioneered its use were so impressed by the ability of the drug to dampen down emotion and psychotic thinking that they used the term 'pharmacological lobotomy' to describe its mode of action.[7]

The Phenothiazine drugs as a class were first used in 1934 to attack urinary infections and as insecticides; in other words, for the purpose of pest control. They continue to be used for eliminating communications from interpersonal pests. In the ten-year period from 1955 to 1965 over fifty million people were given these drugs. Needless to say since 1965 this figure has become considerably higher.[8]

The American psychiatrist, Henry L. Lennard, and his associates consider that the restraint of communication is one of the major hazards of using psychotropic drugs. They call attention to the fact that psychotropic drugs tend to inhibit the different modalities of communication. Thus, tranquillized patients tend to gesture less (kinesic modality) and to lose inflection and tone of voice (para-linguistic modality). One might also add that these people have less to say (linguistic modality) because they find it so hard to think.[9]

Their own research proves this point. Using groups of three people, Dr Lennard and his co-workers studied the effects of a moderate dose of Chlorpromazine in comparison to that of a placebo. They found the tranquillized members of the group were much less active and that in terms of communication, they tended to be ignored by the non-drugged members of the group.[10] The implications of these results include the possibility of new psychiatric problems arising in children of chronically tranquillized parents.

Given that drugs are used to punish and restrain and that they can cause dangerous new physical and emotional syndromes, the question arises whether their disadvantages outweigh their advantages. Perhaps the first consideration is that there are disadvantages as well as advantages in drug therapy. Most people do not take this into account when taking or prescribing today's superabundant medicinals. Too many doctors and relatives of patients are so concerned with quieting a patient that they think this end result is worth almost any risk.

The answer to this question must be a matter of personal value. If one sees man as a machine and despair as a manifestation of this machine going wrong, then it is not illogical to choose mechanistic means in order to eliminate the alleged malfunction. Since practitioners consider despair to be a biochemical abnormality, they choose biochemicals to deal with the problem, and if the new biochemicals themselves cause damage, they refer to this damage as unfortunate aspects of a necessary process of biochemical readaptation. However, if one sees man as a sentient being, capable of change and choice as to his personal relationships and social organization, then it is illogical to take a cavalier attitude towards a treatment which can lead a person to be less capable of feeling, choosing or changing.

Ideally, no drugs should be used at all. Problems arising from confused, constricting or destructive relationships can best be alleviated by providing an alternative relationship in which one person compassionately and empathetically attends to another's fears and despair. Regrettably, experienced therapists and places where this process of 'listening with the third ear' can take place are few and far between. Therefore, additional aids are often required.

Drugs can be a help in psychiatric practice, but not as they are generally employed. Their sole function should be as an adjunct to social intervention, never as a treatment in and of itself. Their principal benefits have to do with enhancing communication and rapport among a group of people which includes someone in distress. This may seem paradoxical because I have already pointed out the many ways in which drugs can decrease communication. However, this side effect is not an absolute consequence of drug therapy, but stems from the wrong drug being given to the wrong person at the wrong time.

If we consider the predicament of the man who saw dinosaurs, it is clear that it was not he who should have been sedated, rather his wife, his neighbour, his boss and his doctor. Perhaps it would not have been necessary to sedate all four, just two or three people of those who were actually upset would have been enough to calm everyone down. Then all the people might have had a second think about whether they really had anything to be upset about.

It has long been known that doctors or nurses prescribe drugs because they themselves are anxious and upset, but the treatment is given to someone else. Dr Thomas Main, of the Cassell Hospital in Surrey, has described this situation in an article entitled 'The ailment'.

Perhaps many of the desperate treatments in medicine can be justified by expediency, but history has an awkward habit of judging some as fashions, more helpful to the *amour propre* (self-esteem) of the therapist than to the patient. The sufferer who frustrates a keen therapist by failing to improve is always in danger of meeting primitive human behaviour (revenge) disguised as treatment. I can give one minor instance of this. For a time I studied the use of sedatives in a hospital practice, and discussed with nurses the events which led up to each act of sedation. It ultimately became clear to me and to them that no matter what the rationale was, a nurse would give a sedative only at the moment when she had reached the limit of her human resources and was no longer able to stand the patient's problems without anxiety, impatience, guilt, anger or despair.

A sedative would alter the situation and produce for her a patient who, if not dead, was at least quiet and inclined to lie down, and who would cease to worry her for the time being. (It was always the patient and never the nurse who took the sedative.)

After studying these matters the nurses recognized that in spite of professional ideals, ordinary human feelings are inevitable, and they allowed themselves freedom to recognize their negative as well as their positive feelings that had hitherto been hidden behind pharmacological traffic. They continued to have permission to give sedatives on their own initiative, but they became more sincere in tolerating their own feelings and in handling patients, and the use of sedatives slowly dropped almost to zero. The patients, better understood and nursed, became calmer and asked for them less frequently.[11]

Another example is provided by the 'snow phenomenon', a term coined by Dr W. S. Appleton, to denote the massive overdosing of patients. He studied the records of twenty-five people who had been 'snowed' with over 1500 mgm. of Chlorpromazine per day. He found that the use of such large doses directly correlated with the inexperience and anxiety of the attending doctor.[12]

The problem of treating the doctor or nurse is more difficult because everyone expects them to be more knowledgeable than they are and not to share the general public concern about sex or aggressiveness. Perhaps a good rule for any hospital emergency room would be that no person is given a psychotropic drug without the prescribing physician being given at least an equal amount! It would be preferable for the more inexperienced house officers to be sedated before being asked to see any psychiatric patients. In that way they might find it easier to speak with them and discover what was bothering them. Surely the widespread use of Chlorpromazine since the mid-1950s has been of most benefit to the professional people who prescribed it. It is true that many patients who have been treated with Chlorpromazine are either out of hospital sooner or not sent to a long-stay custodial care hospital as they might have been before the fifties. However, the number of admissions per person seems to have increased, a situation that has become known as the 'revolving door'.

The change in duration of hospitalization may have little to do with the direct effects of the drug on the patient, but rather may indirectly reflect a less anxious attitude on the part of the psychiatric professionals towards those whom they are supposed to help. In other words, because they are more tolerant of the deviant behaviour and experience of their charges, the doctors and nurses do not feel the need to be as controlling of the lives of these people as had previously been the case.

To be less controlling of others does not mean that the others are going to get out of control. That depends on the attitude, and in particular, the level of anxiety of all the people concerned. A more tolerant attitude can permit a less heavy-handed approach towards those who, under pressure of internal or external stress, have entered a psychotic, manic or depressed state. 'Common sense' no longer dictates that people have to be dragged away from their problems or from their alternative states of reality. On the contrary, it is psychologically necessary for people to work through the psychosis or depression and, if help is requested, the first and most essential task is to establish a rapport with them. In order to accomplish this, the therapist must be able and willing to consider a shift in his own consciousness.

In some instances both parties to a therapeutic encounter can rise to the occasion without any biochemical aids. In others drugs can facilitate the encounter. In either case, the need is for the patient and therapist to shift their consciousness up or down in order to meet at a mutually agreeable level. Then they can be of use to each other, perhaps just by listening. Let me illustrate both situations.

A friend referred a young West Indian actor to me. John had several years' history of manic episodes which had resulted in several hospitalizations and treatment with tranquillizers, Lithium and ECT. When I came to know him he had been appearing in a West End stage play. One day during the middle of the play he picked up a chair, threw it towards the audience while screaming obscenities, and stomped off the stage. Afterwards he went to stay with some distant relatives and proceeded to drive them up the wall by staying up all night and by insisting they talk with him or feed him at all hours of the day or night.

The usual course of treatment for someone in this state would be to have him admitted to hospital and given a course of Lithium. If he responded, well and good, otherwise he might also be given ECT. In either case, the cycle of mania and treatment would continue to occur and the young man would be left with little insight as to what his mania was all about. Alternatively, one could try to make contact with him while he was in the manic state, and by talking with him help him to come down.

I chose the latter way and indirectly, via a person I had known for a long time and who had had a history of mania himself. Robin had been an Oxford don and published some brilliant work in mathematics before becoming a well-known drop-out. At this particular time he was working for a service called BIT, answering the phone and providing a community information service. I discussed the problem with him and asked him if he would be willing to meet the young actor. Robin agreed.

John went to the BIT office where Robin engaged him in non-stop conversation for five hours. In the evening both returned to the home of John's friends where they had a meal and talked throughout the night. In the morning John went to sleep for the first time in several days. Robin slept near him on a mattress on the floor.

When he awoke the next day, John was still high, but obviously beginning to come down. Again he went to the BIT office where he continued his manic dialogue with Robin for many more hours, till he became so exhausted he begged to go home. There he snatched a sandwich and afterwards fell into a deep sleep until the middle of the following day. He awoke feeling refreshed. His state of mind had completely changed and he was no longer manic, although he could remember most of what had happened since the incident at the theatre. Two weeks later he was back at work.

This is not an example of interpersonal heroics. Robin knew how to engage a person like John and help him through the manic state he had entered. Others could do likewise, by taking a stimulant or by achieving a similar state of mind on the basis of their own experience and ability to shift into another level of consciousness without the use of drugs.

In another situation, a colleague of mine was seeing a young man, Richard, who was depressed and suicidal. Although he had been in psychotherapy for several years and had made some progress in exploring the reasons for his depression, he remained very discouraged about the course of his life. A crisis occurred at the approach of his twenty-first birthday. No amount of discussion seemed able to convince Richard that he could ever break his ties with his family and, in his words, 'grow up'. So he had decided to shoot himself.

My colleague thought that if Richard could surmount the crisis he would have a good chance to complete his therapy and make something of his life. But he also realized that Richard had entered such a forlorn and hopeless state that his suicidal intentions were quite serious. So he proposed to his patient that he desist from committing suicide till the stroke of midnight on the day of his birthday, and that twelve hours prior to this time, both he and the young man take a small amount of LSD. He told his patient that this drug would not just make him high as other stimulants had done, but produce a lateral shift in his consciousness such that he might find alternative reasons for remaining alive. He said that he would also take some of the drug, so as to be able to talk with him on his own terms if he wanted to do so. My colleague emphasized that if after the appointed time he still wanted to commit suicide, he would not try to deter him.

The meeting passed uneventfully. Richard sat very still throughout most of the experience, only occasionally breaking the silence with a laugh. At midnight, an alarm clock rang. Richard looked up, smiled and thanked his therapist for staying with him throughout the day. He no longer intended to kill himself. Years later he remarked that the significance of that day centred about the intensity of the silence in the room. Never before had he communicated so well with another person; never before had he felt so understood. It gave him the courage to continue in therapy and work through his hostility to and dependency on his family, both of which were at the root of his depression.

When, as in this example, drugs serve to heighten awareness, rather than decrease it, when they enhance communication rather than hamper it, then their use may be justified. Even in favourable circumstances, however, it is best to be circumspect about taking or prescribing drugs, because it is easy for biochemical intervention to be abused. Yet it is possible to establish guidelines in order to ensure that the risks attendant in the administration of drugs are minimized.

1. Psychoactive drugs should only be given in small doses and for a short period of time. Any drug which is given in any other manner is being misused. This means that the use of long-acting tranquillizers like Modicate should cease. The fact that drugs like Modicate are invariably prescribed with another drug in order to counter their severe side effects is an indication of the obvious dangers of this form of treatment.

2. Drug intervention does not have to be limited to the diagnosed patient. It can be directed towards any member of the relevant social network including patient, relatives, friends or therapist.

3. Either sedatives or stimulants may be employed depending on the state of mind of the different members of the groups.

These guidelines take into account the social as well as physical sequelae of drug therapy. Large doses indicate a failure of communication with or understanding of the patient by his therapist. Prolonged doses indicate a loss of interest. One can try to avoid either situation by taking the trouble to find out which members of the family or group are fuelling someone else's distress. These people may not be the most distressed, or in obvious distress at all. Such individuals are the fulcrum for others' ups and downs. A small change at the centre of the social seesaw can mean that large changes will take place elsewhere in the network. Moreover, the nature of the change that would best be introduced into a group is not always immediately clear, and this also needs to be correctly assessed. It is not a simple matter of giving a tranquillizer to whoever occupies the social centre and letting things die down in the knowledge that when one member of the group is drugged, all the others will be affected. In some circumstances it would be most helpful to employ a mental stimulant in place of a tranquillizer. There may even be occasions where a tranquillizer might be prescribed for one person and a stimulant for another.

However, these guidelines should not be seen as an excuse for expanding the use of drugs in the name of social intervention. If a correct assessment of the interpersonal forces that generate a psychiatric event can be made, and if sufficient communication can take place between therapist and whoever is in distress, then drug treatment may hardly be necessary.

Notes

1. *Contemporary Psychology*, 19, no. 1 (January 1974), p. 9.
2. Richard Hunter and Ida Macalpine (eds.), *Three Hundred Years of Psychiatry 1535–1860* (London, Oxford University Press, 1963), p. 1031.
3. Conolly, *The Treatment of the Insane without Mechanical Restraints* (London, Smith, Elder & Co., 1856), quoted by Hunter and Macalpine, *Three Hundred Years of Psychiatry*, p. 1032.
4. ibid., p. 1033.
5. ibid.
6. *American Medical News*, 22 July 1974. This advertisement by Sandoz Pharmaceuticals is typical of drug adverts.
The ethical and practical side effects of promoting psychotropic drugs have been discussed by Robert Seidenberg, 'Drug advertising and perception of mental illness', *Mental Hygiene*,

55, no. 1 (January 1971), pp. 21–31; Mike Gravel (U S Senator), 'Corporate pushers', *Playboy* (September 1972), pp. 142–3; and Henry L. Lennard *et al.*, *Mystification and Drugs Misuse: Hazards in Using Psychoactive Drugs* (New York, Perennial Library, 1971).

7. P. Huegenard and H. Laborit, *Journal de Chirurgie*, 67 (1971), p. 631, discussed by Lennard *et al.*, *Mystification and Drugs Misuse*, p. 83.

8. Murrey E. Jarrik, 'Drugs used in the treatment of psychiatric disorders', *The Pharmacological Basis of Therapeutics*, 4th edn, ed. L. Goodman and A. Gilman (New York, Macmillan Co., 1970), p. 155.

9. Lennard *et al.*, *Mystification and Drugs Misuse*.

10. L. J. Epstein, B. G. Katzung and H. L. Lennard, 'Psychoactive drug action and group interaction process', *Journal of Nervous and Mental Disease*, 145 (1967), pp. 69–78.

11. *British Journal of Medical Psychology*, 30, part 3 (1957), pp. 129–45.

12. 'Snow phenomenon', *Psychiatry*, 28 (1965), pp. 88–93; quoted in Lennard *et al.*, *Mystification and Drugs Misuse*, pp. 29–30.

3   ECT: The Slaughterhouse Discovery

I certainly am in a strange state. Early last week I suddenly came to – so to speak – and wondered where I was and how I got there. I learned that I had had something called 'electric-shock treatment' that had caused me to lose my memory. Now I know how Eve must have felt, having been created full grown out of somebody's rib without any past history. I feel as empty as Eve.

It was all very peculiar, I was puzzled – but only vaguely. I really felt too vague to care. Nothing really bothered me. Not at first. I felt physically very well. I felt vegetabilized and calm. I didn't have enough memory to think, or even worry, with. And then, because the apartment was so familiar, my mind seemed to open a little, and my memory began to come back. I mean my memory for where I was – for simple, household things. Although there were odd gaps even there. I remember my first morning at home. I thought of breakfast, and I turned to Alan [her husband]: 'What do I usually have for breakfast?' He looked a little startled, but he told me – an egg and a cookie.

The hospital had told me to take it easy, to rest at home for a few weeks, not even to think about my job. I knew where I worked, and that I was an economist and analyst. But it was no problem not to think about my work. Work was something that drifted across my mind from time to time. It didn't interest me. Any more serious reading – a book that required any background of general knowledge – I simply couldn't read. I couldn't understand it.

ECT: The Slaughterhouse Discovery

I went back to work one Monday morning and up to my office and sat down at my desk, and my old associates flocked around. Most of them looked familiar, and I was able to remember some of the names. I was still feeling pretty good. Then I started going through my desk – all the current papers and pamphlets and so on. I gathered that I'd been working on the income of security dealers – relating their earnings to the gross national product. The papers were full of professional terms that seemed familiar. I knew what they were, but I didn't know what they meant.

I came home from the office that first day feeling panicky. I didn't know what to do. I was terrified. I've never been a crying person, but all my beloved knowledge, everything I had learned in my field during twenty years or more, was gone. I'd lost the body of knowledge that constituted my professional skill. I'd lost everything that professionals take for granted. I'd lost my experience, my knowing. But it was worse than that. I felt that I'd lost myself. I fell on the bed and cried and cried and cried.

But you know how it is. One always hopes, or tries to hope. I told myself that maybe it was only a matter of time. If I was patient, maybe in time everything would come back to me. So I went back to the office determined to try. I was going to start all over again. But mostly it was discouraging. There weren't just gaps in my memory. There were oceans of blankness. And yet there seemed to be a kind of pattern. My childhood recollections were as strong as ever. That, I've gathered from my reading about electric shock, is quite typical. The fog of amnesia increased as I came forward in time. The events of the past several years were the blurriest and the blankest.

But the worst of all my problems was that I couldn't seem to retain. I couldn't hang on to my relearning. Only a part of it. The rest kept sliding away again.

So I did what seemed to me the only sensible thing. I applied for disability retirement. I asked for one concession. I asked to be allowed to stay on – without pay – as what's called

59

a 'guest employee'. They were kind enough to grant both my requests. I have my retirement, and I also have a desk at the office. I go there almost every day. I can type. I can do low-level clerical work. And I'm trying, still trying, to rebuild my mental capital.

Electric-convulsive therapy – E C T electroshock – is one of the more refined physical treatments which comprises the psychiatrist's armamentarium. It is widely employed as an adjunct, or alternative, to sedatives and tranquillizers in situations of severe emotional upset. In current practice the procedure is clean, quick and simple. The patient is made comfortable on a bed. A short-acting barbiturate and muscle relaxant is given intravenously. After he has fallen asleep and his muscles have become totally flaccid, electrodes are placed on either side of the skull and an electric current of about 80–120 volts is applied for 0.2 second. After about an hour or so the patient will awake in a confused state, often with a headache, but also unaware of whatever had been bothering him. The procedure may be repeated six to twelve times during an average course of treatment.

The psychiatric literature generally considers E C T to be devoid of serious side effects. This uniformity of opinion seems to reflect the lack of definitive research as to the short or long term disadvantages of E C T. It also doesn't take into account the viewpoint of the many articulate people who have undergone this form of treatment. Mrs Natalie Parker, a thin attractive woman in her early fifties, is one such person. I have begun the chapter with excerpts from her detailed description of the effects of E C T, as related by her in an article in the *New Yorker* magazine by Berton Roueché.[1]

Mrs Parker became depressed after orthodontic work on her gums left her cosmetically disfigured. On the advice of a psychiatrist referred to her by her family doctor, she entered mental hospital where she was given a course of electric shock. Afterwards she felt fine for a few days, but then, as she became more aware of the gaps in her memory, she became very agitated and depressed. It was as if her mind had become as damaged as her body. For her this was an even greater disaster because her very identity and way of life had been dependent on her ability to think.

Mrs Parker was fortunate. After a period of intense despondency about her loss of intellectual facilities she was able to adjust to her new situation. This adjustment was helped by a probing curiosity about the effects of E C T on friends, neighbours and acquaintances. She discovered that permanent memory loss was a very common feature of the treatment, but that this side effect was often overlooked. Only because she was a professional woman with a specialized and demanding job, was she forced to confront the massive amnesia that followed E C T. Otherwise she might have believed that the treatment had left her 'perfectly whole and complete'.

Neither shock nor electric-shock therapy is a recent innovation. Over 1,900 years ago, Pliny the Elder (A.D. 23–79) recommended the application of the live torpedo-fish (electric ray) for easing headaches as well as the labour of a woman about to give birth. The famous physician, Galen (A.D. 201), stated, 'The torpedo-fish has such stupefying power that, being touched with the spear by the fisherman, and the quality passing from the stick up to the hand, it suddenly renders him stupefied and asleep.'[2]

Prolonged bloodletting was a more common procedure for various mental maladies. It could and did lead to a literal state of shock (circulatory collapse). If people survived it was noted that they often returned to a different state of mind.

I Haven't Had to Go Mad Here

Throughout the Middle Ages and up to and including the present day, the systematic application of terror has been a basic method of forcing a person back into sanity. Among the techniques that have been utilized are the sudden plunging of an unsuspecting patient into a lake from a room with a trap-door device, the burning of the scalp with boiling water, and the sudden pouring of ice-cold water over the naked body. The former dunking technique was highly favoured and elaborate apparati were devised in order to allow and regulate the submersion of the patient under water. Regrettably many of these people drowned.

In 1725 the English physician, Patrick Blair, put forward the 'Cataractick way of cold Bathing'. This consisted of the pouring of a measured quantity of cold water from a measured height onto the head of a blindfolded patient. Blair pointed out that this technique was a great advance over the hazards of dunking. He also detailed the following additional advantages:

1. The Surprise upon being blindfolded ... is a great means to the recovery of Reason.

2. Tho' at a second operation there is no more a surprise yet the Terror of the former creates such a dread and horror of it (as) much contributes to produce the desir'd effect.[3]

Blair detailed his treatment of a married woman whose symptoms consisted of neglecting her wifely duties and refusing to talk. She had not responded adequately to prior treatments which had included 'frequent bleedings, violent Emeticks, strong purgatives and potent Sudorificks and Narcoticks'.

The woman was blindfolded and stripped. The nurse and attendants then forcibly lifted her and tied her down to a chair which was placed in a bath tub. Cold water was poured on her head while the doctor repeatedly questioned her as to whether she would be willing to return to her husband and family. After thirty minutes she finally agreed. The water was stopped and the lady was put to bed with a sedative. But the next day she refused to return home. So she was again bled and given emetics and purgatives. A week later the water treatment was repeated, but this time an additional pipe was added so that water could be squirted into her face and other parts of her body as the doctor thought necessary. After sixty minutes, she agreed to return to her husband and love him. But again, the next day, she recanted. A third treatment over ninety minutes was given and the same happened.

By now the doctor was feeling sorely tried. So he threatened the woman with another course of water. He had her stripped, blindfolded and ready to be put in the chair when,

being terrified with what she was to undergo she kneeled submissively that I would spare her and she would become a loving obedient and dutiful wife for ever thereafter. I granted her request provided she would go to bed with her husband that night, which she did with great cheerfulness ... About one month afterwards I went to pay her a visit, saw everything was in good order ... Being thus successful I was willing to know the pondus of water and the pressure her strength was able to undergo ... By ... calculation it appeared that in ninety minutes there was fifteen ton of water let fall upon her ...[4]

The scientific respectability of this treatment was assured because the amount and force of the water used could be readily quantifiable. The dosage – how much water and how often applied – was determined by the persistence of the patient's symptoms and his or her continued refusal to act 'normal'. A similar situation exists with electroshock.

A further parallel can be drawn from the fact that both

treatments require repeated applications. The first shocks generate the fear and anxiety which then motivate the patient to change in order to avoid any future shocks. In this regard Blair is explicit, and a recent study by the New York psychiatrist, Alfred Gallinek, came to the same conclusion. He has demonstrated that the fear and anxiety that accompany electroshock increase with the number of treatments.[5]

Other popular remedies included the Rotary Machine, which whirled the patient round and round like a test tube in a centrifuge, and further variations of cold water showers or douches. These procedures often resulted in 'shivering-fits'. Therefore they can be considered the forerunners of the modern convulsive therapies. Shock therapies so impressed Benjamin Rush, a humanist, signer of the Declaration of Independence and one of the founders of American psychiatry, that he had a special cell built for new patients at the Pennsylvania mental hospital where he worked. It had an iron grating above it, and in the ceiling above the grating and in the ceiling above that. The medical attendant could then douse his patient with cold water from a height of one, two or three storeys.[6] Rush also favoured inducing fits by drilling a hole in the back of his patient's neck and allowing it to suppurate.[7] Other physicians would incise the front of the skull and stick peas inside the wound in order to produce a similar effect.

Benjamin Franklin was a colleague of Rush who was also interested in the treatment of the insane. Following his famous experiment with kites and lightning in which he was knocked unconscious and suffered a brief period of amnesia, he suggested 'trying the practice on mad people'.[8] In fact, in the eighteenth century the medical use of electricity had shown a marked revival. Static electricity machines had replaced the torpedo-fish, and by the 1750s the Leyden jar – an early battery – began to be used extensively for the relief of nervous disorders. John Birch was a well-known London surgeon, and founder of the electrical department of St Thomas's Hospital, who used to treat his melancholic patients by passing electric shocks of varying intensity across the skull. These shocks, however, were limited by the size of the battery which was at his disposal. It is not likely that they produced a grand mal seizure as in the case of E C T.

This was to come about two hundred years later. The German psychiatrist, Manfred Sakel, had been treating people addicted to morphine with small doses of insulin. He noticed that sometimes they went into a deep coma and that his results were better when this happened. As Sakel was also interested in people who had been diagnosed as schizophrenic, he began to apply his method to them. Aside from the coma that was induced, patients treated in this way often developed grand mal seizures which could be successfully controlled by the intravenous injection of glucose.

Paralleling the work of Sakel, the Hungarian psychiatrist Meduna began to use camphor oil and the drug Pentylenetetrazol (Metrazol, Cardiazol) to induce grand mal seizures in his schizophrenic patients. He thought that there existed an antagonism between epilepsy and schizophrenia. Meduna reasoned that the way to cure schizophrenia was by inducing epilepsy by artificial means. (It has since been demonstrated that epilepsy and schizophrenia are not mutually incompatible.) Moreover, from the standpoint of those who advocated a strong dose of fear along with whatever else was done to the mental patient, a further advantage of this method is that the patient is gripped by agonizing fear and panic once the drug has been injected and before the seizure begins.

Yet both procedures suffer from similar disadvantages. They require intensive nursing and medical care. They should not be employed in the case of patients with many kinds of prior illnesses. And they can and have resulted in severe injury and death.

At about the same time that Sakel and Meduna were developing their respective treatments, the Italian psychiatrist Ugo Cerletti was endeavouring to induce grand mal seizures in dogs by sending a 125 volt current through electrodes applied to their mouth and rectum. He had also adopted the methods of Sakel and Meduna in treating his schizophrenic patients.

Naturally Cerletti also thought that electricity could be applied to men as a convulsive stimulus. But he had many problems with his canine experiments, including the death of several animals after relatively low voltage currents had been delivered to them.

By 1937 Cerletti was still ambivalent about the possible use of electric shock in humans. On the one hand he thought that the method would be safe if the technique was correct, but on the other hand he was aware

of the terror with which the notion of subjecting a man to high-tension currents was regarded. The spectre of the electric chair was in the minds of all and an imposing mass of medical literature enumerated the casualties, often fatal, ensuing upon electric discharges across the human body.[9]

Cerletti didn't feel able to proceed and was depressed in the face of his inactivity. Then a colleague of his, Professor Vanni, informed him that at the Rome slaughterhouse hogs were killed by electricity. Cerletti decided to investigate the methods used at the slaughterhouse in order to settle in his mind, once and for all, the dangers of applying electricity to man or animals. In various papers Cerletti describes how his visit to see the hogs killed led to the development of electroshock therapy.

I went to the slaughterhouse to observe this so-called electric slaughtering, and I saw that the hogs were clamped at the temples with big metallic tongs which were hooked up to an electric current (125 volts). As soon as the hogs were clamped by the tongs, they fell unconscious, stiffened, then after a few seconds they were shaken by convulsions in the same way as our experimental dogs. During this period of unconsciousness (epileptic coma), the butcher stabbed and bled the animals without difficulty. Therefore, it was not true that the animals were killed by the electric current; the latter was used, at the suggestion of the Society for the Prevention of Cruelty to Animals, so that the hogs might be killed painlessly.

It occurred to me that the hogs of the slaughterhouse could furnish the most valuable material for my experiments. And I conceived, moreover, the idea of reversing the former experimental procedure: while on dogs my aim had been the use of minimal quantity of current capable of inducing a seizure without harm to the animal, I now desired to establish the time, duration, voltage and the method of application that would be necessary to produce the death of the animal. Electric current would therefore be applied through the skull, in different directions, and through the trunk for several minutes. My first observation was that the animals rarely died, and then only when the duration of the electric current flowed through the body and not through the head. The animals that received the severest treatment remained rigid during the flow of the electric current, then after a violent convulsive seizure, they would lie on their sides for a while, sometimes for several minutes, and finally they would attempt to rise. After many attempts of increasing efficiency, they would succeed in standing up and making a few hesitant steps until they were able to run away. These observations gave me convincing evidence of the harmlessness of a few tenths of a second of application

67

through the head of a 125 volt electric current, which was more than sufficient to insure a complete convulsive seizure.

At this point I felt we could venture to experiment on man, and I instructed my assistants to be on the alert for the selection of a suitable subject.

On 15 April 1938 the Police Commissioner of Rome sent a man to our Institute with the following note: 'S.E., 39 years old, engineer, resident of Milan, was arrested at the railroad station while wandering about without a ticket on trains ready for departure. He does not appear to be in full possession of his mental faculties, and I am sending him to hospital to be kept there under observation . . .' A diagnosis of schizophrenic syndrome was made based on his passive behaviour, incoherence, low effective reserves, hallucinations, deliriant ideas of being influenced, neologisms.

This subject was chosen for the first experiment of induced electric convulsions in man. Two large electrodes were applied to the fronto-parietal regions, and I decided to start cautiously with a low-intensity current of 80 volts for 0.2 seconds. As soon as the current was introduced, the patient reacted with a jolt and his body muscles stiffened; then he fell back on the bed without loss of consciousness. He started to sing abruptly at the top of his voice, then he quieted down.

Naturally, we who were conducting the experiment were under great emotional strain and felt that we had already taken quite a risk. Nevertheless, it was quite evident to all of us that we had been using a too low voltage. It was proposed that we should allow the patient to rest and repeat the experiment the next day. All at once, the patient, who evidently had been following our conversation, said clearly and solemnly, without his usual gibberish: 'Not another one! It's deadly!'

I confess that such explicit admonition under such circumstances and so emphatic and commanding, coming from a person whose enigmatic jargon had until then been difficult to understand, shook my determination to carry on with the experiment. But it was just this fear of yielding to a superstitious notion that caused me to make up my mind. The electrodes were applied again, and a 110 volt discharge was applied for 0.2 seconds.[10]

A typical grand mal seizure followed the second shock. Cerletti and his colleagues 'held their hearts in their mouths' as the man went rigid, stopped breathing, became pale, then cyanotic, and finally emerged from the convulsion with a deep snoring breathing and spasmodic muscular movements. Eventually the man awoke, looked about and asked what had been going on. Cerletti considered this to be a sign of his success as previously the man refused to talk with him.

Another fourteen shocks were delivered to this person, who, most aptly, can be called Cerletti's 'guinea-pig'. Having become more communicative, the man was discharged from hospital and electroshock (Cerletti's term) treatment was born.

As with my discussion of drugs, essential questions arise as to the use of electroshock. Why is it so popular? What does it do? Whom does it benefit?

Again, the answer does not lie with the patient alone, rather in the way the E C T mediates the interconnected needs and wishes of the patient as well as his or her family, doctor and larger social milieu.

In the first place, E C T was developed because Cerletti and his colleagues wished to effect a cure for people who had been labelled as 'schizophrenic'. These patients tended to be most refractory to treatment, hence they constituted a tremendous challenge to the psychiatric profession, especially before the advent of tranquillizers.

The enthusiasm which greeted E C T reflected the conscious needs of the psychiatrist for help in dealing with extremely frustrating individuals. If the latter seemed to respond to E C T with socially appropriate behaviour, I would suggest that they were, in the main, responding to the interest and optimism of their doctors, rather than to the voltage delivered across their temples. It is now well known that schizophrenic patients will respond to any new treatment, whether vitamins, sugar pills, or holding hands, so long as the attending doctor is interested in it. As soon as the interest fades, then the patient tends to relapse. That this happened with E C T can be clearly seen from the fact that the treatment seemed to lose its efficiency after its initial period of development, when the initial enthusiasm had faded away – and after E C T had been superseded by tranquillizing drugs; in other words when the enthusiasm was directed elsewhere. However, for many psychiatrists, E C T still represents the next step after drugs if the 'schizophrenic' persists in his disturbing behaviour.

Aside from schizophrenia, E C T has been applied to a wide range of psychiatric problems, from obsessional states to paranoia, from hyperactivity to hypochondriasis, from anti-social behaviour to depression. At present E C T is most widely employed against depression.

The severely depressed individual is someone racked with guilt, shrunken with self-pity, withdrawn and uncommunicative. Unable to feel the underlying murderous hostility to family and friends, this person tends to lie back and indulge in hopelessness and helplessness. The end point is often physical exhaustion or suicide. The effects of E C T on such people and their families and doctor, illustrate many of the reasons, explicit and implicit, why the treatment continues to be used.

Empirically, depressed people sometimes demonstrate a

rapid recovery. At one moment they may be tearful and un-able to cope, and later, after a few shocks, they may be up and about, working, and carrying on the normal (i.e. non-depressed) relationship with family and friends.

The patient is pleased because she, as is most likely, or he, feels better without having had to take the trouble to find out why she felt bad in the first place. The family is pleased because it is functioning again. Beneath the façade, all sorts of interpersonal time bombs may be ticking away, but for the moment they can be ignored. The doctor is pleased because his self-image as an all-powerful healer has been confirmed. Furthermore, if the treatment has been done privately he has made a considerable amount of money.[11] Finally, 'Society' is pleased because one of its members is back at work and not a drain on the taxes.

Alternatively, the patient may not respond to E C T at all, or may only manifest a partial remission of symptoms. Then a further course of E C T may be given. This also tends to happen in the former case, because even when the initial treatment is 'successful' relapses are likely within a few weeks or months. A total of fifty to a hundred shocks are not uncommon, and it has been known for a patient to receive as many as one thousand shocks over the course of his treatment lifetime.[12]

E C T seems to work by inducing a retrograde amnesia.[13] In essence the patient is buying a period of time during which he cannot remember what is bothering him. Consequently, he is less inclined to behave in a manner calcula-ted to bother others. But this only partially explains the in-fluence of E C T.

As a procedure E C T is invested with magic and fantasy. The apparatus of anaesthesia, the small black box covered with dials and buttons, the electrodes attached to the head, everything is charged with significance for both patient and professional staff. The results of treatment are dependent upon the ways in which these people interpret this magic and respond to their interpretations and fantasies.

The most fundamental interpretations of E C T have to do with life and death. As Cerletti described, by the flick of a switch the patient is brought close to death, and then slowly emerges back to consciousness. Cerletti was overcome by emotion because for a while he was not sure whether he had become the angel of death or the harbinger of life.

E C T is the closest that many people come to the experience of death before actually dying. And this is what they want: to destroy the disturbance inside themselves, to kill off the 'bad' and be left with the 'good'. This fantasy explains why some people who are acutely suicidal seem to be helped by E C T. Having had the vicarious experience of suicide, they no longer feel impelled to kill themselves. In fantasy it has already happened.

The desire to kill off despised parts of the self may be so strong that a person may seek shock after shock. Not infrequently his family will collude with, if not encourage, this longing for psychological annihilation. As for the attending doctor, he is not at all displeased to execute various parts of his patients' psyche. In fact, Cerletti's colleague, Bini, coined the term 'annihilation', to describe his method of delivering many shocks to certain patients each day as a means of ridding them – and him – of their disturbance.

Allied to the wish for death is the wish to be reborn. The expectation is that the annihilation of consciousness is but a prelude to the emergence of a new self. E C T plays a most contradictory role in relationship to these hopes. On one hand it is often prescribed in the case of regression in order to prevent the regression. I use 'regression' to describe those occasions whereby people give up previous ties, 'go down' to return to the unconscious self and become like a child in order to be nourished, fed and protected anew. Either the individual who has embarked on this journey becomes frightened and decides to terminate it, or his family and friends get frightened, as well as angered by the intense demands made on them. Yet, the very means chosen to stop the regression gives the impression that it is being allowed to happen. Both in the case of chemical and electrical shock, the patient is given intensive nursing care. He is put to bed. He is put to sleep. He wakes up and is given further care and attention. Shock therapy so provides the excuse for surrogate mothering that it has been called 'regression therapy'.

Shock-induced regression is an illusion. A little care is no substitute for the support required by a deeply regressed individual. The annihilation of consciousness is no alternative to self-understanding and the long process of working through complex psychological issues.

Far from being a means of self-renewal, ECT is an ally of self-hatred. By acquiescing to ECT, a person is permitting himself to be punished for wishes or fantasies ((often associated with dependency, sexuality or murder) which generate intense feelings of guilt. This guilt can be so overwhelming that he will literally do anything to get rid of it. Therefore a terrifying treatment which mimics the experience of death will be very satisfactory for those who see death as the only suitable punishment for their 'crimes'. Similarly, a terrifying loss of mental facilities, akin to a psychological mutilation or castration, may also be seen and appreciated as a just punishment. In either case, the alleviation of depressive, psychotic or other symptoms can be directly attributed to a marked diminution in guilt. Moreover, the amnesia induced by E C T also helps in that the patient may not only forget why he has felt guilty, but may also forget how to express the guilt that remains.

Of course, this 'cure' is only effective so long as the guilt has been alleviated. As the reasons for the guilt still remain with the person, it will gradually build up again and many of the old symptoms will return. Then a second go round may be necessary. But there is usually a limit to the number of times that the treatment can fool the patient's super-ego. When that limit is reached, then there will be no significant diminution in guilt and no concomitant alleviation of symptoms.

What I find remarkable in such situations is the position of the psychiatrist. Invariably he sides with the patient's conscience. Perhaps this arises because we live in a culture in which the overt expression of intense emotion or extraordinary states of reality is severely proscribed. The patient breaks a fundamental, albeit unspoken rule of human relationships in expressing his feelings openly or in a bizarre manner. Therefore he must be controlled and punished. Both are accomplished through the medium of electric shock. Having forgotten what was on his mind, the patient can no longer pass unwanted communications, which often turn out to be the truth about the way the family is functioning, to husband, or wife, or mother or father. And being frightened of further treatments, he may no longer want to do so. In no way can this use of E C T be considered curative. It is just an exercise in social deception.

The more the psychiatrist becomes an arbiter of social and moral rules, the more E C T becomes a tangible expression of power – as compared to the fantasy of power – by the strong, represented by the family and the State, over the weak, the patient. Here, the professional person acts as an agent for the family or the State and thereby assumes the mantle of power on their behalf. All who are striving for autonomy, sexual expression and justice then become subject to his consent. E C T provides the means whereby he withholds his consent and exerts his power. The 'therapeutic efficacy' of the treatment is simply determined by the extent to which the patient will acknowledge this power and subordinate himself to it, or will endeavour to resist it.

I have had the opportunity to witness this use of E C T on a number of occasions. One was at a large mental hospital in the north of England. After years as a staid old 'bin', a new superintendent was attempting to reform the social structure of the place. The ancient staff resisted tenaciously. One of their members, an elderly doctor, tried especially hard to stem the tide of alleged permissiveness. She could not see why the men and women patients should have meals together (although not at the same table), should frequent the same recreation room at the same time, and should be allowed to work together. Nose forward, shoulders stooped, she would slink about the grounds searching for evidence that the chronic cases in her charge had behaved improperly. Anyone she suspected was put to bed, given high doses of tranquillizers, or put on the shock machine. All it took to do someone in was a vague rumour, like 'Mrs X has been seen to light a fag end for Mr V'. Poor Mrs X wouldn't be seen again for a week.

During my stay at the hospital I began to make the rounds of the chronic wards. I soon became familiar with many of the long-stay patients. Among them were a nice middle-aged man and woman, both of whom had been in hospital for over thirty years each, the man for reasons forgotten and the woman for epilepsy. They had not been discharged because they had nowhere else to go. Over the course of the summer this couple began to spend their free time together. During the mid-week socials they would meet and chat and light fag ends which each had found for the other. In the eyes of the hospital gossips they were 'going steady'.

One evening while passing through the recreation room I noticed that they were holding hands. It was a poignant scene. I stopped and watched for a while, exchanged a few words with them, and left. Next morning I noticed that they weren't at breakfast, then lunch, and only the man appeared at dinner. He looked morose. I went over, said hello and asked about his friend. He was very non-committal and reluctant to talk. Surprised, I happened to mention this to a nurse later on in the evening, who casually recalled that the woman had been sedated and put to bed on doctor's orders. Tomorrow she was to receive electric shock. I demanded to know why. The nurse replied, 'An attack of epilepsy.' This made me very suspicious. In the first place the patient hadn't had a seizure in over twenty years. In the second place, E C T is not the treatment for epilepsy – in fact, it is contra-indicated. So I began to nose about, trying to discover what had happened. It was a very difficult task. The doctor in question was nowhere to be found. The nursing staff was tight-lipped and frightened. Eventually I traced the 'seizure' to the fact that the old doctor had caught the old lady with her friend's hand up her skirt. Yet nobody else in a room full of people had seen the same thing.

The woman received her E C T. Days later I saw her and her friend together again walking down a corridor. I stopped them and asked what had really happened. Nothing much. The doctor had just caught them holding hands.

A young student from Sussex University provides a

further example of the political ends to which E C T can be put. Kate was twenty years old and reading history when she fell in love with a radical American sociologist. This resulted in her leaving Sussex in order to help him with his work in London. Her comfortable Surrey family were very upset by her leaving university and were vehemently opposed to her living with the sociologist. But she insisted, and mother and father retreated to the occasional phone call begging her to come home.

About a year later, during a holiday in Morocco, the man announced to Kate that he wanted to return to the States and didn't want her to come along. She became hysterical, and he had to arrange for her return to England. Mutual friends brought her to Kingsley Hall, a former community in the East End of London where people in emotional crisis could come for help and to live as an alternative to mental hospital.[14]

When Kate arrived she had a dazed look about her. She would sit talking softly to herself but would talk with others if spoken to. During her stay she seemed to oscillate from being as regressed as a small child to behaving as a normal woman. She spoke with her family, told them what had happened and that she was quite content to live at the hall till she felt completely well.

One day her parents appeared at the door and asked her to come with them. She refused. They insisted, pulled her into a waiting car, and took her to the local police station. A short time later the community got a card from the station. It was Kate. She wanted someone to come and take her back to the hall. One of the community promptly responded.

A few days later, the episode was repeated. But this time her sister, a trained nurse, came for her. She did not make the 'mistake' of taking her to the police station. Against her will she was taken directly to a leading London teaching hospital where she was put to bed and immediately given a course of electroshock treatments. The community discovered what had happened because, after days of worrying about her, she rang up from the hospital and asked for help. When they tried to do so, the hospital refused to allow her to use the phone, refused her any visitors aside from her family, and refused to discuss her case with anyone.

Months later I was walking by Primrose Hill when I saw Kate standing on the corner near the park. She looked confused. I ran over and said hello. She looked at me and asked me how it was that I knew her. She didn't know who I was. She was standing on the corner because she had found an old notebook at home with a list of names and addresses in it, and she was trying to visit the people and places in order to understand how they had come to be in her notebook. I looked at the book. All the names were names of her friends. All the addresses were places at which she had lived or visited often. Now all that remained with her was a vague recollection that they had figured in her life somehow. I asked her how she was feeling. She said very well, thank you. Her mummy had told her that she had had several courses of E C T which had helped her very much. She was now living at home and going to the pictures nearly every day. Then she stopped talking, looked about apprehensively and announced that she had to go. It was getting late and mummy expected her home for tea.

What happened with Kate is an example of the exercise of social control in the guise of medical care. Kate, a vibrant, engaging young woman, was treated against her will with electroshock at the behest of her family and with the aid and encouragement of a psychiatric institution. As a result she was robbed of her subjectivity and turned into an amorphous personality, a child, a toy, an object to be manipulated at will by her family. The E C T was the agency by which she was punished for exercising her autonomy, and by which her family demonstrated its power over her. The whole procedure took place with the tacit consent of the State which allowed its medical institutions to be used for familial, political purposes and which did not provide any effective legal redress for either the girl or her friends, once treatment had begun.

There are many parallels between Kate's situation and that of the engineer whom Cerletti first treated. The man had been a complete stranger to Cerletti, as was Kate to the consultant psychiatrist. Both were turned over by one State institution – the family or the police – to another – the psychiatric hospital. Both were given a treatment for which neither had given or been asked for permission.

There are many other complications that result from electro-convulsive treatment. Memory loss is the most obvious one. Perhaps because it is also a means to the patient's symptomatic improvement, it has not been considered a major hazard of the treatment. The amnesia is usually retrograde; that is, extending back over a period of months, years or even decades prior to the E C T.[15] It may also be anterograde; that is, progressing coincidentally with the passage of time and the stream of experience. When they occur together, as just after the patient regains consciousness, the result is extreme confusion. This confusion tends to pass after a few hours, but the amnesia concerning the period before treament may be permanent. Other large gaps of memory may last for months or remain permanently.

The psychiatric textbooks report no loss of intellectual facilities.[16] This can hardly be the case with professional people who suffer both anterograde and retrograde amnesia, as with Mrs Parker, who was not only unable to do her previous work but was also not able to study and retain what she learnt. So we must consider a loss of intellectual facilities to be another potential danger of E C T.[17]

Physical effects are legion. In the days before muscle relaxant drugs were used, upwards of a third of all patients suffered compression fractures of the dorsal vertebrae.[18] Fractures of the arm, leg, pelvis and dislocation of the jaw were not infrequent.[19] Nowadays these fractures are rare, but the muscle relaxant drug, Succinylcholine, carries a risk of its own, which includes prolonged cessation of breathing, apnea, cardiovascular collapse and histamine shock.[20]

Two other major complications tend to be mentioned in textbooks. They are cessation of breathing and cerebral vascular damage. Pin-point haemorrhages may appear throughout the brain tissue. All parts of the brain are vulnerable; ten per cent of all E C T deaths are directly due to intracerebral damage.[21] There is no reason to believe, as some authors have claimed, that all of this damage is reversible.

Many other damaging and detrimental effects of E C T have been described in the medical literature. I am indebted to Dr John Friedberg who has reviewed this literature and extensively discussed these adverse reactions in his paper, 'Electroconvulsive "Therapy" '.[22]

After E C T profound cardiovascular changes have been noted. First there is a slowing of the heart and hypotension, followed by a quickening of the heart and hypertension.[23] E C T deaths have resulted from cardiovascular collapse, damage to the heart and rupture of the heart.[24]

In women, amenorrhoea is common.[25] Both in men and women the endocrine system and body chemistry is affected by E C T; studies have shown an increase in seventeen keto-steroids, S C O T, and phosphate and potassium.[26]

As might be expected, the electrocardiogram (E K G) and electroencephalogram (E E G) are widely altered after electroshock therapy.[27] The latter may take months before returning to normal.[28] In some cases E C T can produce a permanent epileptic disorder in a previously healthy individual.[29]

Considering the actual and potential damage that electroshock can do, one might expect that most doctors would be cautious in prescribing it for their patients. This is not the case. Ever since it was introduced into psychiatry in the late 1930s, E C T has been enthusiastically and uncritically applied to a vast number of people. Surely this is a tribute to the ability of E C T to satisfy the emotional needs of the psychiatrist. But the fact that E C T has survived for so long is not a proof of its effectiveness as a treatment.

There has been a serious lack of rigorously controlled double blind studies of E C T (double blind trials are the standard way of differentiating a non-specific placebo or magical effect, from a specific, active therapeutic influence).[30] On the contrary, there exists a substantial body of work which seriously questions the value of E C T. In one study in which fourteen different psychological tests were given to forty-one patients before and after E C T and to a matched group of twenty-six patients without E C T, no significant difference in the rate of improvement was found between the two groups.[31]

Other work has tested the effects of E C T on the very old and the very young. Hamlon compared a group of twelve elderly patients (each over sixty-five years old) who had been given E C T with two equal control groups of people who did not receive E C T. The groups which received E C T showed significant deterioration in dress, toilet, speech and eating compared with the two control groups. In other words, E C T seemed to accelerate senile brain disease.[32] Levy and Southcombe compared the results of E C T on forty-seven juvenile 'schizophrenics' compared to fifty-six untreated patients and found no difference in results. They concluded that E C T does not influence the course of schizophrenia in patients under thirteen years of age.[33]

Recently, Colin Brewer, who is a lecturer in psychiatry at Birmingham University, has described two patients who were given the procedure of E C T, but without the electric shock. The first was an eighty-year-old woman, who appeared to have had E C T at least once and sometimes two or three times each year since its introduction. The precise reasons for her having had E C T in the first place had been lost … but she was a determined old girl who insisted that it did her good, and she usually got what she wanted. 'After two or three treatments, she made her usual recovery and for good measure complimented us on the nicest E C T she had ever had.'[34]

The other person was a man in his fifties. He had been treated with E C T some years previously for depression. Then his depression returned. Anti-depressant drugs were tried and did not work. Brewer did not think that E C T would help him either, but the man insisted on it. Again the man was put through the whole procedure.

Well, he did get better after six 'treatments' and a few months later when the improvement seemed to be maintained, I told him about my deception, explaining that he could attribute the cure largely to his own resources and should think of himself as having been unhappy rather than sick. He was a bit peeved initially, but was soon pleased to be able to look at himself with greater self-esteem because it was all his own work.[35]

In other words, E C T may be just as helpful when the electric shock is not delivered to the patient. Dr J. Easton Jones calls this kind of therapy, 'Non-E C T'. According to a report in the *Sunday Times*, he treated hospital mental patients for two years from a machine that did not work and nobody noticed. Dr Jones recalls that there were 'no complaints from the patients and although I did not see any consultants, apparently they were satisfied with my work'. He points out that the patients seemed to benefit as much from being put to sleep in preparation for the treatment as from anything else.[36]

It is questionable whether artificially induced convulsions are a therapy. There is no conclusive evidence that the convulsions are curative.

For the patient the pain may be alleviated, but the wound continues to fester. The salutary effects of E C T are illusory. They result from coercion, from the procedure employed (as compared to the actual shock), from the magical interpretations of the patient, and from the retrograde amnesia.

The principal benefits of E C T seem to accrue to the doctor. The 'treatment' protects him from the demands of the patient, from his problems, and from his reality. In turn, the doctor acts on behalf of the patient's family and perhaps the whole of society, to protect them from the patient. This is why the psychiatric profession has tended to cast a blind eye towards the harmful effects of E C T and has never given it a proper clinical trial. People tend to deny what is painful, psychiatrists no less than other men. It is very painful for people whose self-image is that of a healer to see themselves being used as agents of social retribution and self-destruction.[37]

I Haven't Had to Go Mad Here

The convulsive 'therapies' should be phased out of psychiatric practices. This would not be difficult if a minimum of attention were paid to the real needs and wishes of all concerned; patients, family and psychiatrist.

If, for example, the procedure of E C T is so important to many patients as a means of regression, then it should be possible to permit the regression to occur, with or without all the paraphernalia of black boxes and electrical gadgets. It is doubtful whether E C T is necessary either as a suicide restraint or an agent of social control.

Notes

1. Berton Roueché, 'As empty as Eve', *New Yorker* (9 September 1974), pp. 84–100.

2. Galen, 'Proprietà dei semplici XI', quoted by Ugo Cerletti, 'Old and new information about electroshock', *American Journal of Psychiatry*, 107 (1950), p. 87.

3. Patrick Blair, 'Some observations on the cure of mad persons by the fall of water' (1725), British Museum Natural History Section, Collection of J. and I. Martyn (Banksian Mss, no. 103); quoted by Richard Hunter and Ida Macalpine, *Three Hundred Years of Psychiatry 1535–1860* (London, Oxford University Press, 1963), p. 325.

4. ibid., p. 328.

5. Alfred Gallinek, 'Fear and anxiety in the course of electroshock therapy', *American Journal of Psychiatry*, 113 (1956), pp. 428–34.

6. Hunter and Macalpine, *Three Hundred Years of Psychiatry*, p. 326.

7. Roueché, *New Yorker*, p. 89.

8. Hunter and Macalpine, *Three Hundred Years of Psychiatry*, p. 535.

9. Cerletti, *American Journal of Psychiatry*, p. 89.

10. Ugo Cerletti, *The Great Physiodynamic Therapies in*

Psychiatry: An Historical Reappraisal, ed. A. M. Sackler *et al.* (New York, Hoeber-Harper, 1956), pp. 92–4. Also quoted in Thomas Szasz, 'From the slaughterhouse to the madhouse', *Psychotherapy: Theory, Research and Practice*, 8, no. 1 (Spring 1971), pp. 64–5.

In another paper where he discusses the same incident, Cerletti gives different figures for the amount of current applied. He gives 70 volts at 0.2 seconds for the first shock and 110 volts at 0.5 seconds for the second shock. (Cerletti, *American Journal of Psychiatry*, p. 90.)

11. A course of treatment consisting of six E C T may cost from $300 to $750 in the United States, depending on whether it is done on an outpatient basis in the doctor's office or in hospital. In the former case the doctor will make the entire amount less overhead. In the latter case the doctor, if he delivers the treatment himself, takes two-thirds and the hospital one-third. If it is done for him, he usually gets one-third, the attending doctor one-third and the hospital one-third. An efficient E C T service can treat 10–12 patients per hour. Each patient may require several courses of treatment.

12. E. Philtine and P. Polatin, *How Psychiatry Helps* (New York, Harper & Bros., 1949), p. 149. Discussed by John Friedberg, 'Electro-convulsive therapy' (1974). Excerpted in *Madness Network News*, 2, no. 3 (June 1974).

13. It should be noted that there is a sharp difference of opinion in the psychiatric profession as to whether the amnesia induced by E C T is the primary agent of emotional change when it does occur. Some psychiatrists insist that the change is brought about by the actual physical effect of the electrical seizure on the brain.

14. The story of Kate's stay at Kingsley Hall is recounted by Mary Barnes and Joseph Berke, *Mary Barnes: Two Accounts of a Journey through Madness* (London, Hart-Davis MacGibbon, 1971), pp. 280–90.

15. Larry Squire of the Veterans Administration Hospital, La Jolla, California, has found that after five treatments,

patients suffered from an impairment of remote memory extending back as far as thirty-five years. (*New Scientist*, 65, no. 930 (2 January 1975), p. 5.) Other physicians believe that very prolonged memory loss may be a manifestation of hysteria rather than the effect of E C T.

16. For an example see Lawrence Kolb and Arthur Noyes, *Modern Clinical Psychiatry*, 6th edn (New Philadelphia, W. B. Saunders & Co., 1963), p. 540.

17. In a recent study of Goldman, Gomer and Templar, patients were tested with the Bender Gestalt and Benton tests ten to fifteen years after E C T. Major deficits were present, which led the authors to conclude that the data 'suggests E C T causes irreversible brain damage'. (H. Goldman, F. Gomer and D. Templar, 'Long term effects of electro-convulsive therapy upon memory and perceptual motor performance', *Journal of Clinical Psychology*, 28 (1972), pp. 32–4).

18. A. Barker, J. E. Barrett and J. B. Funkhouser, 'Spinal injuries in shock and epileptic convulsions', *American Journal of Psychiatry*, 99 (1942), pp. 387–90; Friedberg, 'Electro-convulsive therapy,' p. 3.

19. Kolb and Noyes, *Modern Clinical Psychiatry*, p. 540.

20. Louis Goodman and Alfred Gilman, *The Pharmacological Basis of Therapeutics*, 4th edn (London, Macmillan, 1970), p. 613.

21. J. L. Jacobs, 'The effect of electric shock therapy on cerebrospinal fluid pressure, protein and cells', *American Journal of Psychiatry*, 101 (1944), pp. 110–12: W. S. Maclay, 'Death due to treatment', *Proceedings Royal Society Medicine*, 46, no. 13 (1953); A. Ferraro, M. Helfand and A. Roisin, 'Morphologic changes in the brain of monkeys following convulsions electrically induced', *Journal of Neuropathology and Experimental Neurology*, 5 (1946), pp. 285–308.

22. Friedberg, 'Electro-convulsive therapy', pp. 2–6.

23. M. D. Altschule, 'Further observations on vagal influences on the heart during electroshock therapy for mental disease', *American Heart Journal*, 39 (1950), pp. 88–91.

24. N. Malamud and A. Zheutlin, 'Fatal cardiac complications during electroshock treatment', *Journal of Nervous and Mental Disease*, 117, no. 5 (5 May 1953).

25. Paula S. Fine, 'Women and shock treatment'. Some psychiatrists say that it is the condition that is being treated with E C T that produces the amenorrhoea and not the treatment.

26. H. Hoagland *et al.*, 'Changes in the electro-encephalogram and in the excretions of 17 keto-steroids accompanying electroshock therapy of agitated depression', *Psychosomatic Medicine*, 8 (1946), pp. 246–51; S. H. Mann *et al.*, 'Cerebrospinal fluid glutamic oaxalacetic acid transaminase in patients receiving electro-convulsive therapy and in neurologic diseases', *Neurology*, 10 (1960), pp. 381–90; A. M. Spiegel *et al.*, 'Physiochemical effects of electrically induced convulsions', *Journal of Neuropathology and Experimental Neurology*, 4 (1945), pp. 277–90.

27. S. Bellet *et al.*, 'The electro-cardiogram during electric shock treatment of mental disorders', *American Journal of Medical Sciences*, 20 (1941), pp. 167–77; M. Feld and G. D. Saul, 'The limbic system and E C T seizures', *Comparative Psychology*, 1 (1960), pp. 281–90.

28. F. Boucher and E. Callaway, 'Slow wave phenomena in intensive electroshock', *EEG and Clinical Neurophysiology*, 2 (1950), pp. 157–62.

29. M. I. Assael *et al.*, 'Centrencephalic epilepsy induced by electrical convulsive treatment', *Electroencephalography and Clinical Neurophysiology*, 23 (1967), pp. 193–6.

30. One study comparing effects of E C T in two groups of twenty depressed patients has been done in Edinburgh. One group was treated as usual and the other group also received the usual treatment except that the first two E C Ts were simulated. The authors claim that the group which did not receive the two simulated E C Ts did better than those that did. However, the full placebo effect was not measured. The mean number of treatments per patient which produced an anti-

depressive effect in the first group was 6 as compared to 7.15 in the group which received two simulated E CTs, although two patients of the first group did refuse further treatment. (C. P. L. Freeman *et al.*, 'Double-blind controlled trial of electro-convulsive therapy (E C T) and simulated E C T in depressive illness', *Lancet*, 8 April 1978, pp. 738–40.)

31. Friedberg, 'Electro-convulsive therapy', p. 8; I. W. Scherer, 'Prognoses and psychological scores in electro-convulsive therapy, psychosurgery and spontaneous remission', *American Journal of Psychiatry*, 107 (1951) pp. 926–31.

32. S. Atkinson and J. S. Hamlon, 'Electro-convulsive therapy: a controlled study of its effects in geriatric patients', *Geriatrics*, 11 (1956), pp. 543–8; Friedberg, 'Electro-convulsive therapy', p. 8.

33. S. Levy and R. H. Southcombe, 'Value of convulsive therapy in juvenile schizophrenia', *AMA Archives of Neurology and Psychiatry*, 65 (1951), pp. 54–9; Friedberg, 'Electro-convulsive therapy', p. 8.

34. Colin Brewer, 'E C T: White man's magic?', *New Psychiatry*, 1, no. 5 (14 November 1974), p. 8.

35. ibid.

36. Oliver Gillie, 'Shock for shock cure doctors', *Sunday Times*, 15 September 1974, p. 2. Dr Jones is a pseudonym for a general practitioner who at the time he was giving E C T was working as an anaesthetist.

37. The fault does not lie only with the psychiatrist. Many patients are skilful in enlisting the psychiatrist in their own project of emotional and spiritual annihilation. The rub is that in giving E C T in order to prevent one kind of suicide (physical), he may be helping to bring about another form of suicide (existential).

4 Psychosurgery: 'I Canna Hear the Buggas No More'

The back ward of a Glasgow mental hospital: a row of thirty beds, tightly packed, lines each side of a long, narrow room. Dishevelled, dirty old men lie on the beds staring into space. One, named Michael, yells coarsely:

'Get away ye buggas! Get away ye buggas, damn it! Get away ye buggas! Get away, ye buggas, damn it! Get away ye buggas!'

His screams continue over many months. Neither drugs, multiple electric shocks, nor other physical restraints are able to stop him. Finally, the staff, being driven to distraction, decide that a prefrontal lobotomy is necessary.

Michael is given a sedative and taken to the operating theatre. A local anaesthetic is injected into a tiny area to the side of each eye and about an inch above it. Two small holes are drilled in each place. Blindly, a thin knife is passed through one hole to a depth of two inches, rotated through an arc of thirty degrees and removed. The procedure is repeated on the other side. Almost immediately, Michael becomes disorientated and silent. Later, the screams resume:

'I canna hear the buggas no more! I canna hear the buggas no more! I canna hear the buggas no more!'[1]

Psychosurgery is based on the observation that certain areas of the brain affect mood and behaviour and the assumption that by altering or interfering with the function of these areas emotional disturbances can be controlled or vanquished.

The Portuguese neurologist, Egas Moniz, and his neuro-surgical colleague, Almeida Lima, are generally credited with the first attempts to put these ideas into practice. In 1936 Almeida operated on patients from a state mental hospital. He severed the connections between the front part of the patient's brain (the frontal lobe) and his thalamus, the bi-lateral walnut-shaped structure in the centre of the brain underneath the lateral or temporal lobes.[2] The result is akin to cutting the wires between two major telephone exchanges. Cerebral communication is disrupted on a wide front. Moniz thought that by interfering with communication between the frontal lobes and the thalami he could 'change the paths chosen by the [nervous] impulses in their constant passage so as to modify the corresponding ideas and force thought into different channels'.[3] The operation is called the prefrontal lobotomy or leucotomy and is similar to that performed on Michael.[4]

Moniz and Almeida considered their initial work to be successful because they were able to produce gross changes in the emotional life of their patients and obtain a reduction in certain symptoms. Many of their psychiatric and neuro-surgical colleagues concurred. Soon the operation was performed all over the world, both as originally developed, and in several variations.

One technique consists of the removal of symmetrical portions of the frontal lobes called topectomy.[5] Another widely used procedure is that of transorbital lobotomy. Dr Walter Freeman introduced it to the United States where he and others employed it on many thousands of patients.[6] In this operation anaesthesia is secured by the administration of two electroshocks. Once the patient is in the post-convulsive coma a slender, sharply pointed instrument is inserted through the bony cavity above the eye to a depth of three inches, rotated left and right and removed. Two more electroshocks are given and the same is done on the other side. Freeman claimed that this technique was a great advance because it is easy, takes little time, requires minimal hospitalization and can be done very cheaply.[7]

Concurrently other investigations focused on the area of the brain below and surrounding the thalamus known as the hypothalamus and the limbic system.[8] These areas are of central importance in the control of autonomic responses such as blood pressure, temperature, appetite, sleep as well as stress reactions including fight or flight. Experiments performed on cats and other animals showed that the stimulation of certain of these areas could cause the animal to become intractably violent. Alternatively, cutting of portions of the hypothalamus, the amygdala – bean-shaped concentration of cells comprising part of the temporal lobe – and the cingula – central arched folds of the cerebrum forming the roof or uppermost portion of the limbic system – could lead a vicious animal to become docile and peaceful. Within a short time these experiments were extended to humans in the anticipation that the centre of 'primitive emotions' had been found and that by cutting, freezing (cryosurgery), poisoning (alcohol, olive oil), burning (electrocoagulation) and irradiating (by direct radiation or implanting of seeds of radioactive material) of these areas violent or otherwise unmanageable people could be controlled. Although the idea of a 'violence centre' has proved to be incorrect, the operation of hypothalamotomy, amygdalotomy and cingulotomy have become very popular. Many patients have been pacified by these procedures, to which the term 'sedative surgery' has been applied.

I Haven't Had to Go Mad Here

Recent advances in psychosurgery have led to a combining of procedures and have enabled surgeons to become more selective in the degree of damage they do. Dr E. Turner recommends the combination of cingulotomy, frontal lobotomy and temporal lobotomy for people experiencing rage, fear and depression – a sort of cranial clean-out.[9] The British team Crow, Cooper and Phillips prefer to implant twenty-four to thirty-six electrodes in the frontal lobes which slowly destroy the cortical tissue over a period of several months by passing an electric current through the implanted electrodes. At the same time they utilize the services of a 'psychotherapist' to monitor changes in the personality of the patient and help him adjust to the operation.[10]

Other doctors have implanted over 120 electrodes in different parts of the thalamus, hypothalamus and limbic system. They then slowly destroy these areas, perhaps first stimulating them with tiny electrical currents. Dr Peter Breggin, a psychiatrist and director of the Center for the Study of Psychiatry in Washington, D C, has intensively studied the literature on psychosurgery and points out that it is now perfectly feasible for electrodes to be put into a person's brain and for the brain to be then stimulated or destroyed by remote-control devices.[11] Indeed, Dr José Delgado of Yale University has employed related techniques on bulls, monkeys and human beings, and advocates the widespread extension of these methods for the physical (external) control of the mind.[12]

Yet psychosurgery is not a safe or benign procedure. Immediately after the operation the patient often suffers from vomiting, incontinence, facial asymmetry and convulsions. He may lose muscle tension and become confused and disorientated.[13] Cerebral haemorrhage and swelling are major dangers and significant numbers of people have died as a result of the complications. Other sequelae may be grotesque. Dr Ross Speck notes:

For a time I was assigned to care for post-lobotomy patients on the surgical ward. I can remember a number of these poor souls when infection or increased intracranial pressure intervened and forced the cerebral cortex and underlying brain tissue through the bilateral burrholes, so that it appeared that the person had three- or four-inch horns growing out of his head.[14]

In the longer term the lobotomized person may become grossly obese as a result of increased appetite and, in the majority of cases, he will demonstrate many of the signs of organic brain damage including loss of intellectual facilities, loss of memory, lethargy, silliness, lack of social restraint, diminished emotional responsiveness, regressive behaviour and deterioration of the personality.[15] All this is not surprising as psychosurgery is essentially an attack on normal brain tissue. In ninety-nine per cent of all cases no anatomical, histological, cytological, physiological or biochemical lesion has been found, either during the preoperative examination or from an autopsy. This fact is a basic drawback as some lobotomists would agree. Thus, Freeman and Watts have declared, 'We believe that the chief obstacle to the more widespread employment of prefrontal lobotomy is the absence of any demonstrable abnormality in the brain thus operated upon.'[16]

Paradoxically many neurosurgeons openly acknowledge the damage they do. They say it is necessary to obliterate their patient's capacity for creative judgement, spontaneity and introspection in order to conquer his psychological disturbance. William Scoville refers to lobotomy as a 'blunting operation', and he includes all the newer forms of psychosurgery as 'partial' lobotomies which dull the personality.[17] Needless to say, many of these personality changes are irreversible.

Walter Freeman has estimated that about 50,000 lobotomies were performed in the United States between the late 1930s and 1950.[18] In the next decade the rate of operations tapered off because of the introduction of tranquillizing drugs and a general dissatisfaction with the incidence of side effects accompanying the operation. But since the early 1960s lobotomy has been undergoing a revival and now 400–600 operations are estimated to take place in the United States each year.[19]

In England about 15,000 operations were performed up to 1960.[20] The rate never tapered off and it is estimated that 400 operations a year are still being done.[21] (Given the difference in population between England and the United States, lobotomies are much more frequent in England.) In addition, tens of thousands of people have been lobotomized in Canada, Australia, Germany, Norway, Japan, Thailand, India and other countries.[22]

Lobotomies were first performed on severely disturbed (i.e. very disturbing to others) individuals with a long history of 'mental illness' not amenable to other treatments. They included people who had been diagnosed as schizophrenic as well as individuals who were incapacitated by depression, anxiety and tension because of obsessive thoughts or fears.[23] After the operation, the obsessive thoughts, ideas or hallucinations do not disappear, but, at best, the patients do not seem to be bothered by them.

In their textbook on psychiatry, Arthur Noyes and Lawrence Kolb state:

In general, lobotomy may be recommended after a two-year

illness if the patient has, in the meantime, received active treatment with tranquillizing drugs, insulin, and electroconvulsive therapy without beneficial results.[24]

Note that there is no mention of psychotherapy!

In fact very few patients were subjected to the full range of treatments, including psychotherapy, before being given lobotomies. Certainly in the period from 1936 to 1950 many were long-term residents in mental hospitals who gave trouble on the wards – soiled, screamed or were otherwise uncooperative – and were considered a social nuisance as well as a drain on private and public funds. As Walter Freeman stated in 1971 while speaking about the usefulness of lobotomy in large custodial institutions, 'It proved to be the ideal operation for use in crowded state mental hospitals with a shortage of everything except patients.'[25]

Freeman was especially proud of his operation on Oretha,

a negress of gigantic proportions who for years was confined to a strong room at St Elizabeth's Hospital. When it came time to transfer her to the Medical Surgery Building for operation (lobotomy) five attendants were required to restrain her ... From the day after the operation (and we demonstrated this repeatedly to the timorous ward personnel) we could playfully grab Oretha by the throat, twist her arm, tickle her in the ribs and slap her behind without eliciting anything more than a wide grin or a hoarse chuckle.[26]

Freeman's operation on Oretha anticipated the use of psychosurgery, from the late 1950s onwards, to pacify unruly women, children, black Americans and other people seen as social misfits.[27]

In one of the first studies published by Walter Freeman and his colleague James Watts in 1942, sixty-one patients were women out of a total eighty people on whom they

95

operated. Of these many were treated for depression.[28]

Since 1936 the majority of lobotomies have been performed on women. Psychosurgeons consider that the operation is potentially more effective with women because it is easier for them to assume or resume the role of a housewife. Lobotomized men find it harder to carry on in intellectually demanding work and as a breadwinner.[29]

The cavalier attitude towards women permeates the attitude of psychosurgeons. At the Second International Congress on Psychosurgery in 1970, Canadian doctors complained that because of unfavourable publicity their hospital refused to allow them to operate on men. It did, however, allow them to operate on seventeen women.

The Toronto neurosurgeon, Earle Baker, described forty-four cases, mostly women with personality disorders or neurotic problems. Among his alleged successes was a suburban housewife who was promiscuous, used to run away from home, and was occasionally suicidal. After lobotomy she is described as a faithful partner in marriage.[30]

Children have also become a major object of focus of psychosurgical attention since the diagnosis of 'hyperactivity' or 'hyperkinesis' became fashionable. Freeman and Watts operated on a dozen children from age four to fourteen. They weren't satisfied with their results because none of the children were able to return to a normal home life; however, they were pleased that the children became less aggressive in hospital.[31]

In 1970 O. J. Andy, Professor of Neurosurgery at the University of Mississippi School of Medicine, published a study on thalamotomy – the cutting of the thalamus – as a cure for hyperactive and aggressive behaviour.[32] Many of his patients were children between the ages of seven and twelve. His associate, Marion Jurko, stated that the goal of their surgery was to 'reduce the hyperactivity to levels manageable by parents'.[33] In other words, they were damaging the brain of the children, not for their sake, but for their parents'. This is a very important principle because time and time again where behavioural problems are the issue, lobotomies are performed not for the sake of the patient but for the sake of relatives, institutions and agents of institutions.[34]

Other neurosurgeons in Europe, Japan, Thailand and India have been active in providing lobotomies for children. V. Balasubramaniam of the Government Mental Hospital in Madras, India, is well known in the West for his amygdalectomies which he performs on children, including some under five years of age, described as 'restless'. Balasubramaniam believes that 'Once the intensity of the behaviour disturbances is severe enough, surgery is warranted, and should not be denied merely because the patient is young.'[35]

In Thailand H. Chitanondh operates on the amygdala on the grounds that it is part of the brain concerned with the sense of smell and that many of the children who come to him with behavioural problems also have smell problems.[36] One of his patients was a nine-year-old boy who was unhappy at home and used to run away, allegedly to smell engine oil in cars.

Chitanondh writes:

Chief complaint of an obsessive smelling habit. For two years before admission he had a strong compulsion to smell engine oil ... He would not give any reason why he had to do this. The parents punished the patient but he would not give up this peculiar habit.[37]

He then performed an amygdalotomy because the boy was suffering from olfactory hallucinations. (Chitanondh seemed unable to distinguish between a hallucination and a habit or obsession. The boy, himself, denied that he was hallucinating.) The result was that his young patient no longer runs away from home to smell engine oil.

Japanese doctors have been concerned with disobedient children too. H. Narabayashi and M. Uno of Tokyo operated on twenty-seven children between the ages of five and thirteen who were characterized by

unsteadiness, hyperactive behaviour disorders and poor concentration, rather than violent behaviour; it was difficult to keep them interested in one object or a certain situation.[38]

In the best post-operative cases these gentlemen affirm:

[They] have reached the degree of satisfactory obedience and of constant, steady mood, which enabled the children to stay in their social environment such as kindergarten or school for the feeble-minded.[39]

The use of lobotomy for the purpose of social control becomes especially obvious when one considers the large number of black people who have received this operation in the United States. During the first wave of prefrontal lobotomy in the 1940s and 1950s many blacks were lobotomized because they made up a significant proportion of patients in state mental hospitals who were chronic and often difficult to manage. In the 1960s and 1970s both blacks and whites have become the object of psychosurgical interest because of the use of the operation against drug addicts, alcoholics and for pacifying people with a violent or criminal disposition.[40] As Walter Freeman put it in the *American Handbook of Psychiatry*:

Lobotomized patients seldom come into conflict with the law

precisely because they lack the imagination to think up new deviltries and the energy to perpetuate them.[41]

The California Department of Corrections is one of several state and federal penal agencies which have explored the use of lobotomy. In the early 1970s the operation was performed on three prisoners at the California Medical Facility at Vavaville. Plans were made to greatly expand the programme by the California Bureau of Prisons. However, a public outcry led to the programme being discontinued.[42]

The idea that brain surgery could be successfully employed for the control of violent criminal activities has been most actively promoted by three Boston doctors : William Sweet, Director of Neurosurgery at the Massachusetts General Hospital; Vernon Mark, Director of Neurosurgery at Boston City Hospital; and Frank Ervin, a psychiatrist who has moved to the Department of Psychiatry at the University of Southern California in Los Angeles.[43]

Shortly after the Detroit riots in 1967 these men wrote in a letter to the *Journal of the American Medical Association* that rioting, arson, sniping and assault could be considered an 'illness' caused by 'brain disfunction' not necessarily related to external social problems. They said :

The real lesson of the urban rioting is that ... we need intensive research and clinical studies of the individuals committing the violence. The goal of such studies would be to pinpoint diagnosis and treat those people with low violence thresholds before they contribute to further tragedies.[44]

Subsequently these three men received hundreds of thousands of dollars in federal and local money which enabled them to open a Violence Clinic at Boston City Hospital for the study and *treatment* of violence.[45]

Interestingly, the violence project had the strong support of Mr Elliot Richardson, the former American ambassador to England who had previously held positions of Attorney General of Massachusetts, Secretary of Health, Education and Welfare, and Attorney General of the United States. In 1970 in testimony before the Senate Appropriations Subcommittee, Mr Richardson made it clear that the violence project was well known to him:

I have had several conversations with Dr William Sweet, who is the project director, about this, and I am bound to say I encouraged him to apply to the Department [Health, Education and Welfare] for funds for this. I had hoped at the time to be able to work with him as the Attorney General of Massachusetts on the basis that the state would also contribute some state funding.[46]

The violence clinic lasted nine months and closed down in the spring of 1972 because of public and professional opposition and the cut off of further funds for it. Ervin then made a proposal to the California Council on Criminal Justice to establish a Center for the Study and Reduction of Violence at the University of California in Los Angeles. This had the public support of Ronald Reagan, then Governor. But it too has been turned down.

Drs Mark, Sweet and Ervin remain undaunted. They still hope to obtain further funding for their work on violence. In support of their ideas they point to the book *Violence and the Brain*, in which the authors hypothesize a direct connection between brain diseases and a wide variety of criminal and political violence.[47]

In the book Mark and Ervin claim that amygdalotomy can be seen as a cure for violence. In evidence they cite the work of other surgeons as well as operations they performed on four people. One was a woman who suffered severe brain damage after a temporal lobectomy. She also became very angry and started to attack hospital attendants. The operation stopped that. Another was a young woman named Julia who had her picture in *Life* magazine and was considered a most successful case. She had one operation, got worse and had a second operation, conveniently done because the original implanted electrodes had never been taken out. After the second operation Julia became extremely angry with her doctors and her mother, who had urged her to have the operation in the first place. She insisted on having the electrodes taken out, although doctors dismissed her rage as 'paranoid'. Later she felt better, went out and killed herself. According to Dr Peter Breggin this suicide was not interpreted as the vengeful act of an angry girl, rather as a gratifying result of the operation, based on the notion that she was getting over her depression![48]

A further indication that the operations performed on Julia were not all for the good was provided by a nurse who has known her, both before and after surgery. The nurse wrote :

He [Dr Mark] implanted a couple of electrodes and proceeded to 'burn out' sections of her temporal lobe. The only problem was that her impulsive behaviour did not leave her and she began to deteriorate in front of my very eyes ... She stopped her wonderful guitar playing. She stopped wanting to engage in long intellectual discussions. Suicidal ... I did see pictures of her in *Life* about the time of the riots as an illustration of a person 'before and after' psychosurgery. That article never mentioned her later deterioration, and severe emotional suffering.[49]

Peter Breggin has done an intensive investigation of another man, 'Thomas R.', whose case Drs Mark, Ervin and

Sweet have often cited in support of brain surgery.[50] Thomas was a brilliant engineer and held many patents. He had apparently developed epilepsy as a child but this was controlled by medication. In 1965 he began to have marital problems and had some severe fights with his wife. He agreed to see his wife's psychiatrist who referred him to Massachusetts General Hospital for a neurological examination which eventually was conducted by Drs Mark, Ervin and Sweet. They concluded that Thomas suffered from 'violent rage' and recommended psychosurgery. Thomas did not want this treatment, but eventually allowed implantation of electrodes in his amygdala; he only acquiesced to the destruction of parts of his temporal lobes while under the effects of lateral amygdala stimulation. Mark and Vernon describe how they obtained this consent:

... we suggested to him that we make a destructive lesion in the medial portion of both his amygdalas – that is, in the area where stimulation elicited facial pain and rage. He agreed to this suggestion while he relaxed from lateral stimulation of the amygdala. However, twelve hours later when this effect had worn off, Thomas turned wild and unmanageable. The idea of anyone's making a destructive lesion in his brain enraged him. He absolutely refused any further therapy, and it took many weeks of patient explanation before he accepted the idea of bilateral lesions being made in his medial amygdala.[51]

The doctors continue:

Four years have passed since the operation, during which time Thomas has not had a single episode of rage. He continues, however, to have an occasional epileptic seizure with periods of confusion and disordered thinking.[52]

Obviously the operation was a success, or was it? Drs Mark and Ervin described Thomas as a violent man and paranoid in regard to his wife. In an interview they have also implied that he was psychotic prior to surgery. Yet the psychiatrist he attended before seeing Drs Mark and Ervin only diagnosed him as having a 'personality pattern disturbance', in other words, mild problems, no psychosis.[53]

The major items of violence attributed to Thomas consisted in his throwing cans of food at his wife, who was not hurt, during arguments. Otherwise his rage seemed to be most closely connected with the wish of Drs Mark and Ervin to destroy parts of his brain.[54]

As for paranoia, this had to do with Thomas accusing his wife of being unfaithful to him. In fact, while Thomas was in hospital, his wife filed for divorce and married the man whom Thomas had been concerned about. It would seem that his perceptions about his wife's infidelity were accurate and his anger quite appropriate.

After the operation in October 1966 Thomas remained in hospital many months. In August 1967 he was released in care of his mother. Within weeks he was picked up by the police in a near-by city too confused to care for himself. After a brief period in hospital he returned home. When finally readmitted to a veterans' hospital he was hallucinating, delusional and very disturbed. According to the hospital discharge summary:

... chief complaint of paralysis from the waist down. Patient stated that the origin of the paralysis was because Massachusetts General Hospital were [*sic*] controlling him by creating lesions in his brain tissue by microwave and they had placed electrodes in his brain tissue some time before. Stated that they control him, control his moods, and control his actions, they can turn him up or turn him down.[55]

For the first time in his life Thomas was diagnosed as

schizophrenic, paranoid type. That was in May 1968. A few months later Thomas was 'arrested by police – involved in a fight, very impulsive'.[56] Thereafter, he wandered from state to state, spending his time in various hospitals and always complaining about his brain being destroyed by electrodes. Far from being a cure, the operation had precipitated a psychosis; led to the disruption of his life, socially and economically; led to his repeated hospitalization; and triggered the very same impulsive, violent behaviour it was supposed to have prevented.[57]

Lobotomy is the only medical treatment which has been formally condemned by the Vatican and banned in the Soviet Union. Although it continues to be practised in the West and the Third World, it should be banned in these countries as well, for a multitude of professional, social, political and ethical reasons.

There has never been a matched controlled study on the effectiveness of lobotomy as a treatment. There have been three retrospective studies done comparing patients who had lobotomies with other patients who were in the hospital at the same time for similar reasons but did not have the treatment. In all three studies lobotomy was found to have no beneficial effects whatsoever.[58] R. Vosburg concluded that lobotomized patients had a psychiatrically induced illness in addition to their initial difficulties. He stated: 'In sum, they act as if they have been hurt.'[59]

Theoretically the operation is based on assumptions about the biological basis of mental illness which have not been proved. While it may be that parts of the limbic system are concerned with fright and fight, they are only part of an intricate and integrated cerebral circuitry. A great deal remains to be discovered. No one, for example, has postulated the existence of a guilt centre, although in most personal and interpersonal situations guilt is an important, if not the most important, component of the complex of emotions which lead people to behave in ways that are seen as mentally ill. Lobotomy just destroys ontogenetically primitive brain centres while neglecting the influence of higher cortical functions. As Peter Breggin has pointed out:

The psychosurgeon picks out the symptom that he wants to focus upon, then destroys the brain's overall capacity to respond emotionally, in order to 'cure' the symptom which he focused upon, completely neglecting that he has simply subdued the entire human being.[60]

Furthermore, the psychosurgeons seem to be oblivious to the psychic life of their patients, or their social relationships. Little consideration is given to the patient's fantasy life, except to exterminate it. Envy, jealousy, revenge and remorse seem to be alien concepts. As for the patient's family, if it is taken into account, it is usually because the doctor has allied himself with one or more relatives in order to effect a change in the patient. In the case of Julia, Drs Mark and Ervin seem to have been allied with the mother in convincing the girl to have the lobotomy. In the case of Thomas, the same doctors seem to have been allied with the wife. But why were these relatives so eager to destroy parts of their daughter's or husband's brain? What did the relatives have to gain? What were their personalities like? The doctors never ask. Moreover, why are the psychosurgeons so eager to destroy parts of other people's brains? Could it be that they see something of themselves in these patients? A necessary part of any retrospective study of a lobotomized person should be a psycho-social profile of the relatives as well as the attending neurosurgeons.

Ethically the operation is intolerable. It is a form of cortical mutilation which goes against all traditions of respect for the human person. Not that the medical journals don't take the ethical issue into account. In an unsigned editorial in a 1969 issue of the prominent British publication, the *British Medical Journal*, the writer recommended psycho-surgery for sex offenders because 'castration is open to criticism on ethical grounds'.[61]

But perhaps the most frightening aspect of lobotomy is the political one. The operation is a step along the path to a therapeutic state dominated by technological totalitarianism. That is why it was so disturbing to see widely influential politicians such as Elliot Richardson and Ronald Reagan supporting the operation. Not that they would admit to being in favour of totalitarianism; all they wanted was an effective form of social control for rule breakers. But then who else but people like them determine the rules which cannot be broken? If violence can be called a sickness, so can almost any forms of political or religious or social dissent. Right-wing politicians can decide that urban rioting is an illness; left-wingers, that capitalism is an illness; Arabs that Zionism is an illness, and so forth. Each side is then perfectly liable to apply known technology to wipe out the so-called epidemic of unwanted beliefs or behaviour.

The lobotomy is simply the logical conclusion of increasingly violent attempts on the part of the state and its agents to control and stifle those styles of emotional and social expression which relatives, neighbours and countrymen consider to be repugnant.[62]

These efforts begin with social ostracism (the labelling process) and proceed through biochemical strait-jacketing (tranquillizing drugs) to the electrical assault of the brain (electroshock) and only terminate with the concrete destruction of brain tissue.

Psychosurgery: 'I Canna Hear the Buggas No More'

Lobotomy is equivalent to psycho-social euthanasia. Psychologically, the patient can no longer think abstractly, fantasize freely, or feel spontaneously. Socially, he has been rendered an incompetent, a legal invalid, as well as a functional invalid dependent on others for some or all of his basic needs.

In my opinion the force which motivates these outbursts of socially sanctioned violence is the wish to locate and destroy that which people find intolerable to perceive and accept as part of themselves, their envy, jealousy, greed, hatred, love and so forth.[63] In the old days, these feelings, individually and collectively, were seen as 'the devil'. They still are. Only a hundred years ago Dr Samuel Cartwright was speaking of 'whipping the devil' out of slaves afflicted by drapetomania – the tendency to run away.[64] Only recently Dr Walter Freeman was getting rid of 'deviltries' in law breakers and disobedient children.

The alternative is to appreciate that people's experiences are essentially intelligible and their emotional suffering is potentially productive. What they need is the space, the time and the encouragement to do, to be and to become more than they have previously been allowed. In the next chapters I will expand upon this theme, and show how the Arbours Association in London and other groups enable individuals to come to terms with themselves without having to annihilate their feelings or give up responsibility for their actions.

Notes

1. Based on an account told to me by Dr R. D. Laing who worked as a psychiatric registrar in a Glasgow mental hospital.
2. For a precise description and excellent graphic representation of frontal lobes, the thalami and their connections, see

Frank Netter, *The Nervous System* (New Jersey, Ciba Pharmaceutical Co., 1969), pp. 40, 72.

3. E. Moniz, *How I Came to Perform Prefrontal Leucotomy*, quoted by Thomas Szasz, *The Age of Madness* (New York, Anchor Books, 1973), p. 158.

4. Lobotomy means a cutting of a cerebral lobe. Leucotomy means a cutting of white matter consisting of nerve fibres or axons which carry the nervous impulses. The two terms are used synonymously.

5. L. Kolb and A. Noyes, *Modern Clinical Psychiatry*, 6th edn (Philadelphia, W. B. Saunders Co., 1963), p. 5551.

6. The late Walter Freeman is generally considered to have been the 'Dean of lobotomy' in the United States. He performed thousands of operations and widely publicized this work. He was former Professor of Neurology at the George Washington School of Medicine in Washington, D C, and was the Honorary President of the International Association for Psychosurgery.

7. Kolb and Noyes point out in their discussion of transorbital lobotomy that: 'Although the operation of transorbital leucotomy appears to be relatively simple and does not require the accoutrements of major neurological surgery, most neurosurgeons hesitate about the blind passing of an instrument through the orbit (of the eye) into the brain.' (ibid., pp. 551–2.)

8. Netter, *The Nervous System*, pp. 146–65.

9. Eric Turner, 'Operations for aggression: bilateral temporal lobotomy and posterior cingulectomy', *Transactions of the Second International Congress on Psychosurgery*, ed. W. Scoville (Baltimore, Charles G. Thomas, 1971). Discussed by Peter Breggin, 'New information in the debate over psychosurgery', U S Congress, Senate, *Congressional Record*, 92d Cong., 2d sess., 1972, 118, pt 26: E3381.

10. Jules Masserman, 'Progressive leucotomy', *Current Psychiatric Therapies III*, by R. Cooper, A. J. Crow and D. G. Phillips (New York, Grune & Stratton, 1963). Discussed by Peter Breggin, 'The return of lobotomy and psychosurgery',

U S Congress, Senate, *Congressional Record*, 92d Cong., 2d sess., 1972, 118, pt 24.

11. Breggin, 'New information in the debate over psychosurgery'; Breggin, 'The return of lobotomy and psychosurgery'.

12. 'The amazing Delgado', *Harper's*, 251, no. 1507 (December 1975), p. 121; José Delgado, *Physical Control of the Mind – Towards a Psycho-civilized Society* (New York, Harper & Row, 1969).

13. Other neurological signs produced by prefrontal lobotomy include plateau speech, sweating, blood pressure changes, babinski sign, borborygmus, monoparesis, coma, ocular changes, aphasia, reflex grasping, hemiplegia, frontal ataxia, staggering, fainting, heart changes, intolerance to drugs and hemichorea. (Walter Freeman and James Watts, *Psychosurgery* (Baltimore, Charles C. Thomas, 1942), p. 293.)

14. C. Attneave and Ross V. Speck, *Family Networks* (New York, Pantheon Books, 1973), p. xiii.

15. Many follow-up studies have found severe brain damage and deteriorating states years after the lobotomy. John Dynes, 'Lobotomy – twenty years after', *Virginia Medical Quarterly*, 95 (1968), pp. 306–8; A. Miller, 'The lobotomy patients – a decade later', *Canadian Medical Association Journal*, 96 (1967), pp. 1095–103; A. Moser, 'A ten-year follow-up of lobotomy patients', *Hospital Community Psychiatry*, 20 (1968), p. 381; R. Vidor, 'The situation of the lobotomized patient', *Psychiatric Quarterly*, 37 (1963), pp. 96–104; R. Vosburg, 'Lobotomy in western Pennsylvania: looking backwards after ten years', *American Journal of Psychiatry*, 119 (1962), p. 503.

16. Freeman and Watts, *Psychosurgery*, p. 18.

17. Breggin, 'New information in the debate over psychosurgery', p. E3381; Breggin, 'The return of lobotomy and psychosurgery'.

18. Personal communication, Freeman to Breggin, 'The return of lobotomy and psychosurgery'.

19. Breggin's estimate. He thinks the rate of lobotomy is increasing rapidly. (It is difficult to arrive at an exact figure as

many operations are performed without the surgeon publishing the results.)

20. Estimate by W. Sargent and E. Slater, 'The return of lobotomy and psychosurgery'.

21. John Pippard estimated 400 per year in 1961. 'Leucotomy in Britain today', *Journal of Mental Science*, 108 (1962), pp. 1223–4. The British surgeon Geoffrey Knight has alone lobotomized over 1,000 people, most since 1960. Discussed in 1970 at Second International Congress on Psychosurgery (it is difficult to arrive at exact figures as many operations are performed without the surgeons publishing the results).

22. Breggin, 'The return of lobotomy and psychosurgery'.

23. Kolb and Noyes state that 'the best results are secured in patients who show tension, agitation and distress, depression, worry, emotional aggressiveness, hostility and excited, impulsive behaviour' (*Modern Clinical Psychiatry*, p. 522). This includes practically anyone who would come to a psychiatrist's office, and most others as well!

They also go on to say, 'If the patient is a chronically deteriorated, inactive *hebephrenic* whose affect has been "burned out", little benefit can be expected from the operation.' As Walter Freeman quipped, 'a deteriorated schizophrenic looks and acts the same with or without his frontal lobes'. Quoted by Breggin, 'The return of lobotomy and psychosurgery'.

24. Kolb and Noyes, *Modern Clinical Psychiatry*, p. 552.

25. Walter Freeman, quoted by Breggin, 'New information in the debate over psychosurgery', p. E3381.

26. Walter Freeman, quoted in *Madness Network News*, 2, no. 2 (February 1974). Freeman also described Oretha as '300 pounds of ferocious humanity' and had to put on the demonstration of her docility because the hospital attendants were so afraid of her. (Breggin, 'New information in the debate over psychosurgery'.)

27. Especially since the advent of operative procedures on the hypothalamus and the limbic system, although prefrontal lobotomies continue to be used for that purpose as well.

28. Freeman and Watts, *Psychosurgery*, tables 5, 6, 7 and 8.

29. Breggin, 'New information in the debate over psychosurgery', p. E3383.

30. E. Baker *et al.*, 'A new look at bimedial prefrontal leucotomy', *Canadian Medical Association Journal*, 102 (1970), pp. 37–41.

31. Ruth Breggin, 'Is psychosurgery an acceptable treatment for "hyperactivity" in children?', *Mental Hygiene*, 58/1 (Winter 1974), p. 20.

32. O. J. Andy, 'Thalamotomy in hyperactive and aggressive behaviour', *Confina Neurologica*, 32 (1970), pp. 322–5.

33. Breggin, 'The return of lobotomy and psychosurgery'.

34. At the Second International Congress on Psychosurgery, Dr Andy was keen to point out that he operated on people with behaviour problems, and not psychiatric disorders! He admitted that he could find nothing neurologically wrong in his patients. (ibid.)

35. V. Balasubramaniam *et al.*, 'Sedative neurosurgery', *Journal of the Indian Medical Association*, 53 (1969), pp. 377–381; V. Balasubramaniam *et al.*, 'Surgical treatment of hyperkinetic and behaviour disorders', *International Surgery*, 54 (1970), pp. 18–23.

36. The amygdala is part of the brain which has been termed the rhinencephalon (because of its olfactory connections), the archipallium (because it was one of the first brain structures to evolve) and the limbic system (synonymous with the other two). In fact the perception of smell is only a small part of its function. In man the rhinencephalon is concerned with mediating automatic (visceral) and emotional responses. (Netter, *The Nervous System*, pp. 152–3.)

37. H. Chitanondh, 'Stereotoxic amygdalotomy in treatment of olfactory seizure and psychiatric disorders with olfactory hallucinations', *Confinia Neurologica*, 27 (1966), pp. 181–96.

38. H. Narabayashi and M. Uno, 'Long range results of stereotoxic amygdalotomy for behaviour disorders', *Confinia Neurologica*, 27 (1966), p. 168.

39. ibid., p. 167. K. Sano of Tokyo has reported on twenty-

two cases beginning with the youngest age of four. In his best result there were 'emotional and personality changes: the patient became markedly calm, passive and tractable, showing decreased spontaneity'. (K. Sano *et al.*, 'Postero-medical hypothalamotomy in treatment of aggressive behaviour', *Confinia Neurologica*, 27 (1966), pp. 164–7.)

40. Peter Breggin, 'The second wave', *Mental Hygiene*, March 1973.

41. Walter Freeman, 'Psychosurgery', *American Handbook of Psychiatry II*, ed. S. Arietti (New York, Basic Books, 1959).

42. Allan Brownfield, 'Psychosurgery: Mental progress or medical nightmare?', *Private Practice*, June 1973, pp. 46–50.

The Department of Prisons tried to 'sneak' the programme through the state legislature, but reporters discovered what was going on and traced the identity of one of the prisoners who was found to have suffered significant emotional and intellectual damage. Because of further negative publicity about lobotomy the Federal Bureau of Prisons announced that it will not permit psychosurgery in its planned psychiatric treatment facility at Butner, North Carolina.

43. All three are members of the Neuro-Research Foundation of Boston.

44. F. Ervin, V. Mark, W. Sweet, 'Letter to the Editor', *Journal of the American Medical Association*, 201 (1967), p. 895.

45. Among the grants were $500,000 from the National Institute of Mental Health to start the violence clinic, monies totalling $188,000 from the Law Enforcement Assistance Administration (a branch of the US Justice Department) for studying 'the role of neurobiological dysfunction in individual violence' especially as it relates to the criminal justice system, and $50,000 from the office of the Mayor of Boston to study brain disorder and violence. Joe Hunt, 'The politics of psychosurgery, part 2', *The Real Paper* (Cambridge, Mass.), 13 June 1973.

46. Joe Hunt, 'The politics of psychosurgery, part 1', *The Real Paper* (Cambridge, Mass.), 30 May 1973.

47. F. Ervin and V. Mark, *Violence and the Brain* (New York, Harper & Row, 1970). The authors relate violence to psychomotor epilepsy. In fact, there is no proven link between violence and psychomotor epilepsy nor are people who suffer from psychomotor epilepsy necessarily violent. Furthermore, the temporal lobotomies (amygdalotomies) which they performed in order to stop the violence (allegedly influenced or caused by the epilepsy) did not stop seizures in those who underwent the operation. All that was shown was that amygdalotomy may have a pacifying influence, something that is well known.

48. Breggin, 'The return of lobotomy and psychosurgery'.

49. From a letter to Breggin, quoted in 'An independent follow-up of a person operated upon for violence and epilepsy', *Rough Times*, 3, no. 8 (November/December 1973), pp. 8–10.

50. Thomas R. was a model for Harry Bensen in *Terminal Man* by Michael Crighton.

51. Ervin and Mark, *Violence and the Brain*, pp. 96, 97.

52. ibid., p. 97.

53. Breggin, 'An independent follow-up of a person operated upon for violence and epilepsy', p. 8.

54. ibid. Breggin quotes his hospital chart during a work-up prior to surgery, 'He has never been in any trouble at work or otherwise for aggressive behaviour, never been in jail or a mental hospital.'

55. ibid., p. 9; quoted by Breggin.

56. Note this is two years after the operation and directly contradicts the assertions of Ervin and Mark.

57. In 1968, Thomas was declared 'totally disabled' by the Veterans' administration. In 1971 he was declared a mental incompetent by the courts. During the hospitalizations in the period 1972–3 he became increasingly violent, writing 'murder' on the ward's walls and going around with newspapers, bags, books and other material around his head to protect him from further surgery. For further details of Thomas's case, see the follow-up study by Breggin, ibid.

For an additional critique of the work of Ervin, Mark and Sweet see Breggin, 'The return of lobotomy and psychosurgery'; Breggin, 'New information in the debate over psychosurgery'.

58. G. Kaczanowski and K. G. McKenzie, 'Prefrontal lobotomy: a five-year controlled study', *Journal of the Canadian Medical Association*, 91 (1954), pp. 1195–6; A. Robin, 'A controlled study of the effects of leucotomy', *Journal of Neurology, Neurosurgery and Psychiatry*, 21 (1958), pp. 262–9; R. Vosburg, 'Lobotomy in western Pennsylvania: looking backward over ten years', *American Journal of Psychiatry*, 119 (1962), p. 503.

59. Vosburg, 'Lobotomy in western Pennsylvania'.

60. Breggin, 'The return of lobotomy and psychosurgery'.

61. 'Brain surgery for sexual disorders,' *British Medical Journal*, 4 (1969, pp. 250–51.

62. To realize the violent intent behind the procedure one need do no more than look at the words that psychosurgeons themselves use to describe the operation. Thus, W. Freeman and J. Watts call the prefrontal lobotomy a 'satisfying surgical *attack*' (*Psychosurgery*, p. 9). Egas Moniz said his purpose was to '*annihilate* a great number of associations' and to suppress certain symptomatic complexes by '*destroying* the cell connecting groups' (quoted by Szasz, *Age of Madness*, p. 159) and so forth [my italics].

63. I hypothesize that people who become psychosurgeons lend their technical expertise to the State for purposes of violent social control because the operation gives them the opportunity to annihilate in others (by means of projective identification and concrete action) psychological attributes which they cannot stand in themselves. The patient's relatives collude with the operation for similar reasons. Ergo, the lobotomized patient is an interpersonal scapegoat on many levels.

64. Morton Schatzman, 'Psychiatry and revolution', *Arbours Network*, 8 (1975), p. 6.

5 The Butterfly Man

And there appeared a great wonder in heaven; a woman clothed with the sun, and the moon under her feet and upon her head a crown of twelve stars: and she brought forth a man child, who was to rule all nations with a rod of iron: and her child was caught up unto God, and to his throne. (*Revelations* 12:1, 5)

He was the Lion of Judah and had journeyed to the centre of the earth and back many times. There was much work to be done. He had to redeem the Good and vanquish the Wicked. But his strength eluded him, and having been thrown out of his lodging, he was desperate for a place to stay. So he drove to a small house in a North London suburb where he had been told that refuge might be found.

This man, whose name is John, arrived in the dead of night, dishevelled. He pushed the bell. No sooner had it rung than he wanted to leave. He was put off by the Celtic cross in the window and was frightened by the two people who appeared in the doorway. What if they were in league with the dragons who had previously tormented him with heads of fire and teeth of fury!

The couple, a man and woman, said they had been expecting him and bade him welcome. A room had been prepared for him, and they suggested that he go upstairs to bed. But John ignored them. He dropped to all fours and slowly began to undulate about the living room. He was no longer a lion, not even a small, thin human being, but rather weak and helpless, one of God's lowest creatures.

An hour passed. The man and woman were getting very tired. They had done their best to comfort John, but to no avail. Finally, they insisted that he get up, walk upstairs and get into bed.

Alarmed at their demands, John managed to sit up and reply, 'Don't be silly! Can't you see? I'm a caterpillar! Caterpillars can't crawl upstairs!'

Taken aback, the woman retreated into silence. Then she exclaimed, 'You may be a caterpillar now, but caterpillars become butterflies. You will too!'

The house is a crisis centre run by the Arbours Association. The temporary dwelling places where the Israelites lived in the wilderness after the exodus from Egypt were called 'Arbours' – places of shade or shelter. The Arbours Association is a mental health charitable association in London which aims to provide shelter and safe anchorage for people who have been buffeted by internal turbulence or external disturbance whether in fantasy or in actuality.

For John, Egypt was his parents' home. There he felt enslaved by his mother's messianic expectations of him which contrasted with his father's incompetence. After university, he took a job with a high salary as a chemical engineer, yet he remained tortured by an image of himself that oscillated between omnipotence and impotence. On one hand he saw himself as the son of God, a ruler of nations 'with a rod of iron', and on the other hand he feared that he was a born loser who would never amount to anything.

This conflict became intolerable after his engagement to a beautiful and demanding young woman. He had a dream in which his mother, Winston Churchill and other dignitaries urged him to save the world from destruction. He tried. He wrote letters to *The Times*. He stood for public office. All to no avail. Then his mood changed. He became very depressed. Every object, every person seemed to scream 'failure' at him. He stopped working and started bathing. These were long, extraordinary baths, sometimes fully clothed, sometimes not. For hours John would lie in the water to which he had added soap, talcum powder, toothpaste and bits of old food as well as his own blood, urine and faeces.

Although obsessed with bathing, John could still discern social reality. He was concerned with 'going mad' as well as being seen as 'mad' by others. Therefore, he consulted a member of the Arbours Association who advised him to seek help at the crisis centre. Yet John was reluctant to do so; he didn't want to go to a mental hospital and was suspicious of a place which he associated with a 'mental asylum'. But then his landlord threw him out for being a nuisance, and he was homeless.

Safe and secure in a room at the centre, John relinquished all attempts to appear 'normal'. Instead he immersed himself in a brilliant kaleidoscope of colour and drama. At one and the same time he could see and participate in everything whenever and wherever it was happening. He was God, the room was an observatory, the house was a mountain on top of the world. Then it changed. The room was a whale and he was inside the whale, full of sperm, feeling very strong. It changed again. He was inside an enormous brain, putting it together, creating a new brain of fantastic intelligence. This allowed him to make a space rocket, a cosmic ark designed to save the one hundred and forty thousand good souls that remained on earth.

These waking dreams were unlike dreams because they

were too real, too vivid. After four days, John changed. He put on his clothes, he came down to dinner, and he rid his wastes in the toilet instead of the bed or on the floor. Hesitantly, painfully, he joined the community which had supported him during the period of disintegration.

The rebirth was rapid and uneventful. One week after he had arrived at the centre, John moved out to a long-stay Arbours household. A day later he started a new job as an industrial chemist. Although he hadn't grown wings, his social antennae were sufficiently strong to allow him to function and be appreciated by people whom he had previously avoided.

Even if all the conflicts which had led him to the crisis centre had not been resolved, they no longer tormented him. He could think, he could work, and sexually he could fly.

There are few places where a person can go through a psychotic experience without the restraint of drugs or other physical treatments. The Arbours Association in London is one such place.[1]

It was founded in 1970 by Dr Morton Schatzman, Vivien Millett, Roberta Elzey Berke, myself and others. We wished to give individuals who had been or could become mental patients the time, space and encouragement to confront, rather than escape from their emotional, physical and spiritual problems and to achieve a personal stance which was truly their own. We have now grown to a network of over forty people and sponsor four households including the crisis centre, a low-cost psychotherapy clinic, a training programme and other activities.

Morton Schatzman and Vivien Millett created the first Arbours community in their home. From 1970 to 1975 several men and women lived with them as an alternative to mental hospital. No special provisions had to be made. The community functioned as an extended family, and Morton (Morty) and Vivien were the parent figures. Others, who lived in the house in order to learn more about our approach, helped out with whatever had to be done.

Subsequently we established four communities – the crisis centre in North London and three other households, one each in South, West and North London. For the most part, all the communities are rented from a local council or private individuals. However, in the spring of 1977 and with the help of a private contribution to the group, we purchased a house in North London for a new community. In each case, the cost of rent or mortgage is considerable.

The long-stay communities are run communally and have from seven to fourteen members each. Residents stay as long as they wish as befits a place which is their home. People who come for a short time are considered to be guests or visitors and are accorded the kind of hospitality that anybody might expect when staying with family or friends.

The accommodation is in comfortable semi-detached houses in quiet residential neighbourhoods. The style of life in the different houses is determined by those who live in them and, in the case of the crisis centre, by its special purpose. No one takes on the traditional roles of 'staff' or 'patient' except when newcomers sometimes find it difficult to cease previous practices. Interestingly, residents with professional qualifications, who have come either as helpers or in need of help, are not necessarily accorded the most respect. Instead it may go to someone like John who underwent an intense and unusually vivid death/rebirth experience. Other sources of prestige in the households are personal presence – including the ability to remain unruffled in the face of another's anxiety – psychological insight and experience.

Whenever possible, every resident shares the tasks of cooking, cleaning, shopping and so forth. Those who do not cooperate may be asked to leave by the other residents, not because they are 'ill', but because they are not contributing to the community. In practice the workload is not evenly divided. Those who are regressed or depressed tend to be given special dispensation. But this tolerance does not last indefinitely.

Residents pay for their stay in an Arbours community according to the basic cost of rent, light, heat, Arbours overheads and according to how much special attention they may require – how much room they take up in the womb. Expenses such as food, records, books and so forth are shared according to the needs and wishes of the people in a particular house. The money comes from the residents themselves or their families, from insurance and from grants by local councils. Many residents do not pay the full cost of their stay, and we endeavour to make up the deficit by means of charitable contributions.

In other aspects of their lives the residents are largely autonomous. They choose whether to work (most do), go to school or stay at home. They choose when to eat and what to eat, when to bathe or not to bathe, when to sleep or not to sleep, and whether to sleep with others or alone. There are few rules, and what rules there exist are made by everyone together. Part of living in an Arbours community involves learning what these rules are, and becoming party to decision-making. Because of this we have minimal problems with violence. Violence tends to happen in situations where rules governing people's behaviour are obscure, contradictory or inflexible. Considering the degree of disturbance which some people have brought to the group – fantasies of murder and mayhem – it is extraordinary how quiet and peaceful life is in an Arbours community.

The surface calm covers an intense inner turmoil of which most residents are quite aware. They also know that the Arbours tries to provide as much interpersonal support as may be necessary for them to confront, contain and understand their hatred and despair. One way we do this is by encouraging residents to enter into psychotherapy or psychoanalysis. Another is by encouraging each community to hold regular weekly meetings with an experienced Arbours member when anything and everything is discussed, whether it is buying a new frying pan, the noise from the hi-fi, or agonizing jealousy felt by one of the residents about another.

A third means is by involvement in the Arbours network – all the people associated with the Arbours who have a knowledge of and take an interest in each other's lives. This group includes the residents of the four communities, non-residents like myself and my wife Roberta, ex-residents, and members of the Arbours training programme.

This programme is a three-year course for psychotherapists and social therapists.[2] The trainees, who come from England, Europe and the United States, participate in the work of the Arbours and attend bi-weekly seminars on a variety of subjects including psychoanalysis, communications theory and the sociology of madness. Each trainee is expected to be in psychoanalytic psychotherapy, live in an Arbours community for at least six months and help at the crisis centre. In their third year the trainees see individuals in psychotherapy under supervision in conjunction with the Arbours psychotherapy clinic. In addition, they attend lectures and seminars given for the public as part of the Arbours general educational programme. They may also write for and be involved with the publication of our magazine, *The Arbours Network*. After completing the course, the trainees may join us in expanding activities of the Arbours network either in London or in their home communities.

The entire Arbours network meets on the first Sunday of every month. Each household takes turns at hosting this get-together of the extended family. The meeting serves as a social gathering, a business convention and an occasion for airing personal disputes and problems. It provides the opportunity for old friends to chat and for newcomers to initiate a relationship with others in the network. The closeness of our personal relationships is the key to the way we work. When someone gets upset, he knows that he can swiftly contact another person in the group to help. This contact is person to person, not person to 'role'. A friend, not a stranger, is being called. And if this friend chooses to intervene as a sympathetic parent or therapist, then it is with the tacit understanding that after a brief period the relationship will revert to its former status.

There have been times when the entire network has had to care for a single person. This happened with Matt who called up one day to apply for a job. He had been working as an orderly in a mental hospital, but came to the conclusion that the drugs and E C T were doing more harm than good. He wanted to learn about 'anti-psychiatry'. We thanked him for ringing, but mentioned that we had no jobs available. In fact, we prefer not to have paid therapists at our communities. We have found that experienced residents who had sorted out their own problems and knew everyone else in the group were the best means of immediate support the communities could have. However, we said we would be pleased to meet him and discuss the possibility of his living in one of our houses. Eventually he moved to a Norbury community in the self-appointed role of a helper. Yet it soon became apparent that it was he who needed the help. He stopped going to work, and began to complain that his body was disintegrating and that everyone was persecuting him. The residents spent a lot of time talking with him and trying to help him through his crisis but to no avail. He was too angry with everyone there, and too frightened to see that it was this very anger that was threatening him. Eventually it was suggested that he move to another community and this he did with some relief. Soon afterwards he moved into an old taxi which the Arbours had bought for travelling from house to house. He preferred the solitude of the passenger compartment to a place in the house.

At a network meeting people argued that it was not inappropriate for Matt to live in the back of the taxi. It provided a fine womb-like space perfectly suited to his state of mind and needs. So they arranged for a bottle of milk to be delivered to the taxi once a day and for Matt to be able to take a loaf of bread whenever he wanted from a near-by bakery. In addition, his psychotherapist, Gregorio Kohon, an Argentine psychologist who had recently joined the group, agreed to see him once a day in the taxi.

It would be nice to say that all worked out well. This was not the case. Although Matt spent much of the day in the taxi, he bothered some neighbours by walking down the street with a jerky gait and talking to himself. One day Matt could not be found. He had been picked up by the police and taken to a mental hospital. He was kept there for a long time.

*

Basically, our relationship with the outside world has been good because we have not advertised ourselves as a hostel or a bunch of nutters, just some people trying to live together. The residents struggle to avoid living out any pre-assigned role as 'mental patient' or 'former mental patient'. As they do not see themselves this way, neighbours do not see them this way either. No more noise, nuttiness or nuisance emanates from an Arbours community than from the average urban house.

Still we are aware that there remains a considerable body of public opinion which feels that anything to do with 'mental illness' or emotional distress should be kept far away. Therefore we ask the communities to maintain a low profile. On the whole, this policy has been successful.

The impetus for continuing to develop and expand the work of the Arbours has been the repeated observation that psychotic states are not inherently harmful. They can provide an opportunity for personal growth as well as collapse and chaos. What happens depends, to a great extent, on the attitudes of the person who is experiencing the world in an altered manner and of those to whom he has turned for support. If the latter, whether professionals or not, are frightened by unusual or odd states of mind or patterns of behaviour, then they are likely to interpret these incidents as signs of a 'mental illness' which needs to be treated, that is, stopped. On the other hand, if the psychotic individual and those about him can tolerate and respect what is taking place, events can take a different course and come to a productive conclusion.

The idea that regression – the flight from adulthood into infancy – or psychosis – the flight from accepted reality to an altered state of consciousness – may be a creative experience has been expressed by numerous writers. The distinguished British psychoanalyst, D. W. Winnicott, saw both regression and psychosis (they may occur separately or simultaneously) as the means by which many individuals seek to shed their false fronts in order to reach a new and vital relationship with themselves and the world. Dr Winnicott advocated a greater tolerance of these phenomena which he termed mechanisms of healing and readaptation. Moreover, he suggested that special provisions should be made so that people could be able to complete the breakdown of the old self, once it had started.[3]

The essential observation is that the breakdown is a cyclic event which includes a period of psychic fragmentation leading to a period of emotional reconstruction. The Polish psychiatrist Kazimierz Dabrowski has called this first phase 'positive disintegration'.[4] In many situations he sees it as the necessary first step for the birth, development and integration of the personality. Similarly, the American psychiatrists Don Jackson and Paul Watzlawick regard the acute psychosis as 'a manifestation of growth experience' which may lead to a rapid, long-lasting and successful therapeutic change.[5]

These conclusions are supported and illustrated by the published accounts of several people who have gone through both phases of fragmentation and recovery. John Thomas Perceval provided one of the first and certainly one of the most illuminating of such narratives. Born in 1803, he was the fifth son among the twelve children of Spencer Perceval, the prime minister of England who was assassinated in the House of Commons in 1812. He had a conventional childhood for a young man of his class, and in his teens he was commissioned as an officer with a cavalry regiment, the 1st Foot Guards. During these years as a soldier he was deeply troubled by religious conflict. Early in 1830 he relinquished his commission and became closely involved with an extreme evangelical cult in Scotland. The members of this cult were called Irvinites. They spoke in an unintelligible gibberish which they believed to be the language of a foreign people. But these people found it hard to put up with the increasingly erratic behaviour of Perceval. As a result he left them and went to Dublin. There he slept with a whore and contracted syphilis. Although he made a rapid recovery, he began to be increasingly bothered by voices. Eventually his brother came and committed him to a mental hospital near Bristol. He remained in hospital for over three years, possibly because he came from a socially prominent family who did not want to be embarrassed by him at home. Then, in 1834, he left hospital and took a wife. In subsequent years he wrote his books, had four daughters and lived to a ripe old age.

He describes the onset of his psychosis:

I was tormented by what I imagined was the Holy Spirit, to say other things, which as often as I attempted, I was fearfully rebuked for beginning in my own voice, and not in a voice given to me. These contradictory commands were the cause, now, as before of the incoherency of my behaviour, and these imaginations formed the chief causes of my ultimate total derangement.[6]

The voices continued to torment Perceval throughout most of his stay in hospital. But the pain diminished when he began to realize that the voices did not come from outside himself, rather from inside himself. Moreover, they were not meant to be obeyed literally, rather to be understood metaphorically.

A vision marked the turning-point in his struggles. He

recalled that he was often tempted by the sight of naked women. One day he saw the image of a 'female of great beauty', 'a creature of flames', someone who was married to one of his friends.

She appeared to descend from heaven unto me, when I was lying on the grassy bank in my wretched prison-yard, and uniting her spirit with my person, filled me with comfort. 'Surely,' I thought, 'she is praying for me and her prayers are heard, and her Spirit is living in me.' I was then, perhaps, bordering upon frenzy or upon melancholy madness, *and thus the Almighty condescended to heal by the imagination that which, by tricks on the imagination, he had wounded, broken and destroyed* [my italics].[7]

This waking dream image bears a strong resemblance to the waking dreams that John described while at the Arbours Crisis Centre and which were a prelude to his self-reintegration.

Barbara O'Brien and Mary Barnes have contributed contemporary accounts of their 'journeys through madness'.[8] Like John Perceval, Barbara O'Brien was persecuted by voices, which she called 'the operators', which forced her to do bizarre and disturbing things. She only began to come through the disintegrative phase of her psychosis when she saw that the operators were aspects of her own thoughts and desires.

Mary Barnes went through a profound regression. She writes,

In 1953, when I was for one year in Saint Bernard's Mental Hospital, I got put in a padded cell. I felt so bad. I lay without moving or eating, or making water or shits. They didn't let me die, they tube fed me. I wanted to be looked after; I didn't know then, I do now, that what I was trying to do was get back inside my Mother, to be reborn, to come up again, straight, and clear of all this mess.

Then in 1965 she found two psychiatrists, Dr R. D. Laing and myself, and a place, Kingsley Hall, where she could 'go down and come up again'. For months she lived in a black box and had to be fed with a baby bottle. Then, slowly, she began to 'come up'.

The five years at Kingsley Hall were all my years for therein was held my past, my present and my future. The Nurse, the teacher, fled; the child returned, crept back into the womb, emerged, grew as never before, in body and soul.

Because psychosis is cyclic it has often been described as a 'journey' or 'trip'. Gregory Bateson, the anthropologist, remarks,

It would appear that once precipitated into psychosis, the patient has a course to run. He is, as it were, embarked upon a voyage of discovery which is only completed by his return to the normal world, to which he comes back with insights different from those of the inhabitants who never embarked on such a voyage.[9]

For Bateson the acute psychosis is a vast and painful initiation rite conducted by the self into the self. It is a means by which the ego sheds its skin and is renewed.

Dr R. D. Laing has commented on the mythic or archetypal qualities of this voyage. He sees it as a retreat from all outer concerns into an inner world of space and time completely removed from all usual constraints and prohibitions. The initial phase is a retreat into the 'self', into the 'womb of all things (pre-birth)'. The return is a passage from inner to outer, from regression to progression, sonic time to mundane time, from 'cosmic fertilization to an existential rebirth'.[10]

This 'going into the self' is not a universally accepted expression of madness. On the contrary, there are cultures where the death of the ego and the reintegration of the spirit are an integral part of the ceremonial movement from child to adult or from adult to man of knowledge. In many other places, both past and present, this experience has been deliberately invoked as a means of healing. It was a common practice, for example, in ancient Greece. The sick came from all over the ancient world to seek cures at the temples of Asklepios, Demeter and Trophonius (Zeus), by means of 'incubation'. Literally, incubation means 'lying on the ground'. The initiate was expected to spend a night in a cave, alone, lying on the ground in preparation for a dream or vision that would, in itself, cure him.

The Jungian analyst, C. A. Meier, points out that once the sacred rite had begun, the incubant was, for all apparent purposes, a prisoner of the Gods. They determined how long he could stay, what food or drink he could consume and when he could leave the cave.[11] This concretely expresses the situation whereby in undergoing the incubation, the incubant is putting himself in the hands of his unconscious. He then waits for the appropriate message from the unconscious in the form of a 'right' dream or vision. When it comes, it needs no interpretation and the disturbing symptoms which brought the person to the sanctuary simply disappear.

The true function of the caves or, in modern terms, the retreat, must be to provide an appropriate setting whereby the dis-ease or internal conflict can become personified or expressed in symbols. The priests or guides must at least encourage this process, once it has begun. This was certainly the case at the crisis centre where Sally (resident therapist with Tom Ryan) acknowledged John's experience as a caterpillar, but also, by bringing up the link between caterpillars and butterflies, intimated that he was moving towards a fundamental personal reorganization.

John's choice of symbols was not a coincidence. The life cycle of the butterfly has tantalized the unconscious of men for thousands of years. It personifies the movement from dependency to autonomy, from impotency to potency, from death to rebirth. Associated with these changes, there is a stage where the larva builds a womb for itself, a chrysalis where its tissues liquefy and then re-form into their final shape. This place can be seen to be the sacred cave, the retreat, the crisis centre, the supportive environment, where a man can allow his emotions to liquefy, his ego to disintegrate prior to re-establishing himself as a vital human being.

Dr Bruno Bettelheim has found this metaphor appropriate to his Orthogenic Institute, a centre in Chicago for psychotic children. He comments,

Deep down the patient knows that this place will have to serve as a chrysalis for him if, after a period of dormancy and inner development, he is to emerge a full person.[12]

The entire metamorphosis has been beautifully described in a dream quoted by C. A. Meier in his discussion of incubation. A man found himself running deep into the earth. Far inside he found an ancient cave. On the floor in the centre of the cave there was a human body wrapped in tar-soaked linen bands. It looked as if it had lain there for countless ages.

It was possible to recognize that this mummy – for that was what it looked like – had the face of a man. I recognized that *it was myself*, and I shivered in spite of the great heat, for I thought that now I was really dead. It now seemed to me that I myself passed into the corpse, and I struggled inside it against what seemed to hold me fast, but it was no use. I struggled again and again until at last something gave way. I made a still greater effort and something else gave way. I felt the bonds crack and I struggled violently with all my strength, for I knew I should die if I could not get free; and I had the feeling that I should have to give up the ghost. I was filled with unimaginable terror. Then the corpse burst its bonds with a terrible cry, so that the roof of the cave burst asunder, and I saw the clear sky far above the roof. I left the corpse just as a bird takes wing and flies away, or as a butterfly leaves its chrysalis, and soared up into the dawn.[13]

Not everyone who comes to the Arbours brings with him the drama of a mythic journey or the desperation of a profound regression. It is more common for a man or woman to seek our help for a depression which drugs or shock therapy have not helped and for which he or she does not want to be institutionalized. In addition many people who have had months or years of hospital treatment come to the Arbours in order to terminate their careers as a mental patient.

Does the Arbours succeed? Morty Schatzman points out that this is an irrelevant question: We do no harm, we do no 'cure'. The Arbours is a place where some people may encounter selves long forgotten or distorted. Given time, with luck, they may hear the beating of their hearts and elucidate the rhythm.

Notes

1. The Arbours Association, 38 Berkeley Road, London N.8 (tel. 01–340 7646, or for the Arbour Crisis Centre, 01–450 6896).

2. For more information write to: Mr Andrea Sabbadini. Co-ordinator, Arbours Association Training Programme, 55 Dartmouth Road, London NW5.

3. D. W. Winnicott, 'Metapsychological and clinical aspects of regression within the psycho-analytical set-up', *Collected Papers: Through Pediatrics to Psycho-Analysis* (London, Tavistock Publications, 1958), pp. 278–94.

4. K. Dabrowski, *Positive Disintegration* (New York, Little, Brown & Co., 1964).

5. D. Jackson and P. Watzlawick, 'The acute psychosis as a manifestation of growth experience', *Psychiatric Research Reports*, 16 (May 1963), pp. 83–94.

6. J. I. Perceval, *Perceval's Narrative: A Patient's Account of his Psychosis, 1830–1832*, ed. Gregory Bateson (New York, William Morrow & Co., 1974), p. 32.

7. ibid., p. 308.

8. Mary Barnes and Joseph Berke, *Mary Barnes: Two Accounts of a Journey through Madness* (London, Hart-Davis MacGibbon, 1971); Barbara O'Brien, *Operators and Things* (Arlington Books, 1958).

9. Perceval, *Perceval's Narrative*, p. xiv.

10. R. D. Laing, *The Politics of Experience* (New York, Pantheon Books, 1967), p. 89.

11. C. A. Meier, *Ancient Incubation and Modern Psychotherapy* (Evanston, Ill., Northwestern University Press, 1967), p. 109.

12. Bruno Bettelheim, *A Home for the Heart* (London, Thames and Hudson, 1974), p. 103.

13. Meier, *Ancient Incubation and Modern Psychotherapy*, p. 12.

6 'I Haven't Had to Go Mad Here'

'Look at the centre of the pendant! Follow every swing! Follow every colour! Look carefully!'

The man tried to keep his gaze on a small piece of metal moving back and forth from a silvery chain. He was obviously uncomfortable and found it hard to concentrate. Only his tight trousers, leather jacket, high-heeled boots and a Mexican sombrero covered the all-pervading panic that had gone on for over a week.

Tony was a drummer in a jazz group and had been through bad patches before. All he had to do was play. But this time the fear hadn't gone away. It had got worse and nothing had been able to soothe him. He just sat, curled up on the floor of his small Liverpool flat, and refused to budge. He only responded when someone mentioned mental hospital. Then, out of the corner of his mouth, he hissed an angry 'no!' before resuming a vacant stare. He had 'the horrors' about being separated from his wife, June, and their eight-month-old son, Mark. Finally, an old friend of the family, who had just qualified as a doctor, broke the deadlock. He said that he knew of a place in London where they didn't use drugs and understood people like him. Would he go there? Tony agreed, if June, Mark and their beagle could come, too.

Gregorio spoke with a soft Latin accent while directing Tony to focus on the pendant and relax. He did not think that Tony would enter into a trance. He was too tense. But Gregorio wanted to make the procedure as convincing as possible. The hypnosis was at Tony's request. Although Gregorio had never practised hypnosis before, he decided that it would be a good way to establish a relationship with him.

First, Gregorio asked Sally to go upstairs to the 'hypnosis box' and bring down the special amulet. Sally complied by fastening a large sequin on to a holder and ceremoniously handing it to him. Then she and the others left the room. Ten minutes later Tony exclaimed, 'It's not working, I still feel terrible!'

Gregorio replied, 'Yes, hypnosis is hard with some people. Let's try yoga. Can you get into the lotus position?'

With that suggestion Tony visibly relaxed. He explained that all week long he had been trying to find his 'spot' on the floor. He believed in the teachings of Don Juan: by sitting in the right 'spot' he gained strength and knowledge, but if he moved, however slightly, then he became weak and his enemies could attack him.

Gregorio asked who his enemies might be. Tony fidgeted but remained non-committal. Then his friend Paul and June came into the room. Quick as a flash Tony hunched his back and assumed a position of silence and immobility. Further discussions revealed that Paul and June, as well as Tony, felt tied, both emotionally and socially, into one miserable knot. Paul confessed that he had once been June's lover before she had married, and he still found her sexy. June mentioned that she had married Tony because he really turned her on when he played the drums. Until the baby was born she couldn't think of anything else but since then Tony had become a big drag. He could never let her care for the child without interfering. He was so demanding, worse than their son. She still found him sexy, but only when he was playing the drums. At other times she was consumed with sexual fantasies about other members of the group. In her view, the crisis occurred because the group was threatening to break up and Tony would have no one with whom to play.

Over the next two days Gregorio, Tom and Sally spent many hours with the couple and their friend, trying to untangle the knot. As Tony felt more able to talk with Gregorio, he spent less time at his 'spot'. Gregorio recalls:

I had to be firm with him. He was in an explosive rage, and I had to show him that he was at liberty to get angry with me if he wanted, that he needn't be afraid of his rage, and that I was perfectly able to look after myself ... After a while he was quite relaxed.

The rage was of volcanic intensity and jealous intent. Tony felt no good as a musician – the group was breaking up; as a man – June fancied other men; as a husband – he found it hard to support the family; and as a father – he wanted to be looked after. But he couldn't express these feelings because he was ashamed of his jealousies and needed the support of those who might be harmed by them. So he projected his anger on to imaginary enemies from whom he sought to protect himself.

With Gregorio's help, the need for fantasied safeguards diminished. Tony became more vocal about his feelings and less concerned about Don Juan. Consequently, June relaxed. She spent more time with her husband and was less concerned about the baby and the dog. But Paul became very agitated. He was preoccupied with the idea that Tony would discover that he was paying for their stay. Moreover, he was very disturbed by the sudden realization that it wasn't June he wanted to sleep with, but Tony. Tony's response to these developments was to insist that everyone head for home, four days after coming to the centre. He was angry that no one thought he was 'sick' any more.

Subsequently, we received two letters from June. It seemed that soon after returning to Liverpool, Tony had a 'gig' with another group and was doing well. Paul had gone off to Scotland to practise medicine. And the baby had begun to walk. The crisis had passed.

This account illustrates the salient features of crisis intervention. It is immediate. It is brief. It includes a number of people, not just a single individual. It involves a mixture of practical and interpretative help, and it can stimulate creative developments in the life of a person or family, as well as alleviate distress.

The conceptual basis for crisis work was established by the American psychiatrist, Erich Lindemann, in response to the Coconut Grove nightclub fire in Boston during World War Two.[1] He studied the effects of the fire on relatives of the victims. Lindemann observed that the inability of many of these people to grieve for their loved ones caused a bewildering array of somatic and emotional problems. He realized that these problems were not the signs and symptoms of an 'illness' but the expression of an unsuccessful bereavement. He reasoned that the best way to intervene in such a situation was to help these people engage in the normal process of grieving. The sooner this happened, the sooner they would be able to carry on with their lives. Treatment, as such, was unnecessary.

In 1948, Lindemann and his colleague, Dr Gerald Caplan, started a community crisis service in the Boston area (Wellesley Human Relations Service). The function of the service was to enable members of the community to regain their emotional and social equilibrium when confronted with major threats to their person or way of life. The threats may be situational – moving house, entering school, hospitalization; interpersonal – marriage, divorce, death of a spouse; or developmental – adolescence, menopause, old age. For the most part these are day-to-day occurrences, not extraordinary events. The crisis unfolds when an individual or family sees them as events which are difficult or impossible to cope with. Then, a specific group of tensions may unfold which include generalized anxiety, guilt, fear and depression, and marked feelings of helplessness and hopelessness.[2] In addition there may be gross changes in behaviour, all of which tend to reflect the internal states I have just described. These responses characterize crisis in the same way that the constellation of somatic distress, preoccupation with the image of the deceased, guilt and hostility characterize bereavement. Consequently, Lindemann and Caplan argued that the best way to intervene in case of crisis is not by treating the symptom of the tensions produced, but by helping the person or family to confront and work through the crisis itself. An added bonus is the fact that crises can generate a meta-stable state whereby, for a short period, one's capacity for learning and readaptation is greater than usual.[3]

Of course, all crises are relative to those who are experiencing them. What was a major trauma in the life of John, the Butterfly Man, or Tony, the drummer, might not be a difficulty for somebody else. The difference lies in how realistically the affected person perceives a situation, the degree of interpersonal support he may have, and the depth of his experience of personal resources. Therefore, in a crisis, the tasks of those who intervene include assisting the

137

person or family to achieve an undistorted picture of what's happening, mobilizing supportive relationships, and acting as an auxiliary ego until the person is able to cope for himself.

Although crisis theory has been elaborated over the past three decades, there exist few facilities in which to practise crisis work. In California in 1962 the Benjamin Rush Center for Problems of Living was opened as an autonomous unit of the Los Angeles Psychiatric Service. A few years later crisis intervention replaced emergency detention at the San Francisco General Hospital. In New York a 'Trouble Shooting Clinic' was set up by Leopold Bellak as part of the City Hospital of Elmhurst.

Later, a special unit of the Bronx Mental Health Center was created for crisis intervention among a large poor Puerto Rican population. This unit was followed by the East Tremont Crisis Center which operates from a converted post office and combines crisis work with a day centre and a sophisticated social work facility.

In 1964 Dr Donald Langsley and his colleagues established the Family Treatment Unit at the Colorado Psychiatric Hospital and have been using family crisis therapy as an alternative to hospitalization. The average duration of treatment is about three weeks and generally consists of a home visit, five office visits and several telephone calls.[4] Results of follow-up studies show that people who received this treament were able to work through their crisis with less disruption of their lives than those who were given the standard psychiatric treatment. With crisis therapy people returned to their jobs sooner and were less likely to need hospitalization or rehospitalization. Moreover the cost of crisis therapy was approximately one-sixth that of the hospital treatment.[5]

In London Dr R. D. Scott has initiated a crisis service at

the Napsbury Hospital. As at the Family Treatment Unit a clinical team visits the family at their home in order to provide active reassurance and support and to prevent the family from avoiding its problems by having one of its members labelled as a 'mental patient'.[6]

Other crisis units exist outside the hospital system and concern themselves with particular kinds of crises. Drugs, suicides and runaway children have provided the impetus for 'free clinics', 'hotline' telephones and communal 'crash pads'.[7] The Samaritans are the most successful among these groups. The project was started in 1953 by an Anglican minister, Chad Varah, who sought to befriend people who were contemplating suicide by talking with them on the telephone. Twenty years later this work has expanded to include 17,000 volunteers taking over 100,000 calls per year in England, Scotland and Wales.[8] It may be significant that during this same period the suicide rate in England has dropped dramatically.[9]

The Arbours Crisis Centre was set up to assist people who had entered an alternative state of experiencing reality or who were threatened by sudden and overwhelming emotional distress or who were suffering a breakdown in their social relationships. Although we had been intervening in such situations for several years, we did not have a place where someone could go at a moment's notice. Sometimes no rooms were available at our long-stay communities. More important, members of these households wanted the opportunity to meet and become familiar with potential newcomers before they would agree to share their lives with them. We found that this vetting process, which could take days or weeks, was simply too long in crises where immediate attention and aid was required. Therefore, we decided to organize another community where people would not have to wait.

I Haven't Had to Go Mad Here

We rented a pleasant comfortable suburban house for the centre. It was agreed that Tom Ryan and Sally Berry would live in the house and serve in the multiple roles of therapist, companion and housekeeper. Unlike our long-stay communities where the social structure was informal and undefined, we decided to maintain clear-cut lines of responsibility and communication at the centre. Our worry was that the delineation of roles would lead to impersonal relationships with those who came to us. This has not proven to be the case; in fact, the opposite has occurred. By living in, Tom and Sally found it easier to establish a rapport with residents and visitors.

The centre opened in January 1973. We made a phone number available (01–450 6896), and from the very beginning we received many calls directly from people in crisis, their relatives and friends, as well as from doctors, social workers and probation officers.

When a call comes in (or letter, which we answer promptly) the resident therapists determine whether the centre can usefully intervene. If not, they try to refer the caller to another and more appropriate agency. For example, we do not try to intervene in case of acute alcoholic intoxication and might refer the person to a hospital or to a branch of Alcoholics Anonymous. If we can help, then an appointment is made to see the person within a few hours and, if possible, at home. We say that a team of people from the centre will be coming to meet the caller.

The team consists of one of the resident therapists, a member of the Arbours training programme and a team leader.[10] The team leader is an experienced psychiatrist or psychotherapist whose function is to assist in the evaluation of the crisis and to coordinate the efforts of the team on behalf of the persons or person in distress.

The crisis team will make the home visit without prior assumptions about who is 'mad' and who is 'ill'. The purpose of the visit is to try to ascertain exactly who is in crisis, who is affected by the crisis and what the crisis is about. This is not necessarily an easy task because individuals and families have a knack of hiding what is troubling them even when they are most desperately asking for help. Yet a home visit can provide infinitely more information about the situation than any number of meetings with single members of the family outside the home.

After the visit the team may conclude that the person who is allegedly in crisis is not the only one but is representing a crisis in the whole family. This often happens when a husband calls up about his wife or the wife about the husband. After meeting them, we may suggest that both stay at the centre together. Even when this is impractical, or only one person stays, we endeavour to hold a regular series of meetings to discuss the difficulties which each partner is having with the other. Some of our most successful work has been carried out in this way with couples while they decide whether to remain together or to separate.

A similar intervention may be called for when a parent phones about an adolescent son or daughter who seems to be behaving in an inappropriate or bizarre manner. After a number of discussions with the family it inevitably transpires that the parents are a great, if not a greater source of disturbance than their child. They may, for example, be going through, yet denying, a mid-life crisis concerned with loss of sexual function, or approaching old age. The affected youngster may be the only family member who is not adept at concealing his feelings.

Dr R. D. Scott of Napsbury Hospital has demonstrated that individuals rarely get admitted to hospitals because they are 'sick', but rather because their position in the family or community has become untenable. He uses the term 'identity warfare' to describe the situation whereby some people become so threatening to the psychic survival of others that their continued presence within the group serves as in incitement to fantasized, if not actual, murder and mayhem. Hospitalization is the means by which the most threatening person, or the one with least power, is sacrificed so that the group identity can remain intact. Or, it may be the means whereby one member seeks refuge from the battle. Alternatively, hospitalization may provide the means for a family member to go on the offensive. By assuming the mantle of mental patient, he or she can make everyone else feel awful.

We try to circumvent these ploys by not immediately inviting the alleged patient to stay at the centre. Later, if it seems useful for someone to become a guest, we may suggest that one or both parents come together with or instead of those who are more overtly upset.

Whatever is done, it is essential to avoid *cultural closure*. This is a term and concept developed by Dr Scott to describe the moment when a person in a family is no longer seen and accepted as a member of the family, but as a stranger, alienated from and by the family. *Closure* is confirmed by the act of diagnosis whereby this person is defined as different and stripped of responsibility for his thoughts, feelings or actions. As Dr Scott points out, once this has happened, and the ex-family member has been handed over to a variety of institutions and their agents for treatment, it is very difficult for the person to regain his prior identity or standing in the family or community. *Cultural closure* exemplifies the issues I raised in the first chapter.

*

The two components of any crisis are the primary issues and the secondary disturbance which follows when the integrity of a person or of a family is threatened. Most psychiatric treatments are concerned with the secondary changes of mood and behaviour. It is rare for people to seek help before the 'crisis syndrome' appears. The admonitions, 'Keep a stiff upper lip!', 'Buckle down!', or 'Work harder!' are deeply ingrained in our culture. People seek outside support only when panic has set in and the guilt, shame and humiliation that attend an 'inability to cope' have become too great. The secondary response is then seen as 'the crisis'. In these circumstances the usual remedies afford only symptomatic relief. They temporarily alleviate the pain while the underlying problems remain unresolved and continue to generate further symptoms.

An added complication is that symptomatic treatment tends to confuse people as to why they are upset. It is not uncommon for someone suffering from depression due to unresolved grief to be told that he has a hereditary ailment or a biochemical aberration. At the crisis centre we work to avoid this complication by making a thorough search for the roots of the crisis. We direct the first stage of our intervention towards enabling people to obtain an undistorted picture of the underlying problems and their secondary ramifications. With some guests sudden realizations have been accompanied by an array of activity which is surprising to all concerned.

Debbie's difficulty was that she had left mental hospital and had nowhere to stay. A social worker had put her up for a few days but couldn't continue to do so. When she came to the crisis centre she was a frightened tangle of tears and thick brown hair which covered her face and blurred her words. For days she remained curled up in a corner,

143

head in her lap, surrounded by the reproachful voices of her long dead mother: 'Debbie, don't do that.' 'Debbie, you ought to know better.' 'Debbie, I'm ashamed of you.'

Then a rapport developed between her and Sally. For minutes at a time she would pull back her hair and tell her about the voices. Sally responded by brushing the hair and trying to untangle it. One Sunday Debbie announced that the hair had to go. It was too long, too matted and too much in the way. Sally agreed and helped her cut it. A maze of constraints went along with the hair. First, she described what was bothering her, a brother who had seduced her and a boyfriend who had left her without seducing her. Later she began to shed her clothes and demonstrate a great sexual interest in everyone about the centre. Finally she stripped naked and took to walking about the house and into the street. Sally eased her back into the house while gently explaining the difference between public and private places.

Debbie stripped in order to reveal a tortured but provocative sexuality. Previously, John (the Butterfly Man) had stripped in order to facilitate his regression. Others have stripped in order to exhibit self-hatred and to solicit punishment. In each circumstance the clothes serve as social metaphors. However, not everyone who comes to the crisis centre has to reveal the naked truth about his fears, wishes or family relationships by divesting himself of his outer garments.

As a rule, the more difficult the guest, the more we call on members of the Arbours to join the team and expand the social network of the person in crisis. Our object is not just to stop the bizarre or disruptive behaviour, but to contain it within a network of sympathetic individuals. This effort may continue for a few days or weeks while we endeavour to be understanding and non-judgemental with guests who are often confused and critical about what is happening to them. It may be necessary to spend a lot of time with them, or leave them alone. We may have to do a great deal of interpretative work, or none at all. The task is how to establish a supportive relationship without becoming intrusive or uncaring. Obviously, someone can't be allowed to do something dangerous, either in or out of the house. But we have found that even the most psychotic person can respond to a clearcut presentation of the facts (like, don't masturbate in the streets because the neighbours won't tolerate it) and will modify his behaviour accordingly.

We don't force anyone to stay in the house, but there are occasions when a guest wanders outside while not realizing how upsetting his state could be to the casual passer-by. Then we ask the person to remain inside until his appearance or actions become less noticeable or less liable to arouse fear or rejection. Sometimes residents wander out and all we can do is walk with them. Fortunately, the neighbours have tended to be tolerant, especially when one young guest, a nurse from New Zealand, who had 'freaked out', rang all the neighbours' doorbells and announced that an atomic bomb was about to go off. On another occasion, this same person screamed and cursed at an elderly Irish lady next door who happened to remind her of her mother. The old lady was taken aback, but Sally, who saw what happened, calmly walked over and explained that the girl was far from home and quite distraught. The neighbour remarked that she could well understand because as a child she had been sent away and become homesick. Instead of complaining about the incident, she came over for a visit with cakes and flowers.

I have often been asked, 'How is it possible for someone

to go through a deep depression or psychosis so quickly? What do you really do at the Crisis Centre?'

The point is that if this experience is indeed a response to a crisis, whether developmental, interpersonal or situational, then the affected person has already entered a state where his personality, his character, his whole life may rapidly change. My task is to assist this change, to enable it to occur as fully and profoundly as possible, not to delay or retard it.

Sometimes this may happen with a person who is already in psychotherapy or psychoanalysis. This was the case with Danny, a forty-year-old American artist who had moved to London after achieving considerable success in New York. Danny had initially consulted me at a time of great unhappiness. His marriage had broken up and he was uncertain whether to paint, sculpt or devote himself to teaching. After several years of therapy the dragon of his self-destruction lay quiet and his work took on a colourful new direction. Then his mother died. She had been the dominating figure in a large extended family. Her death evoked relief and grief, seeming unconcern and a strong attachment to a younger woman who was 'the first with whom I could be openly aggressive and angry'. Then she left him and Danny became distraught. For him this loss confirmed that he could never express his feelings, that his destructiveness knew no bounds, that no relationship was safe. He was convinced that the few friends he had left were plotting to kill him and that I was just waiting for the right moment to get rid of him.

'I'm rubbish, nobody wants me, nobody can stand me. I want to go to mental hospital. I want drugs to put me to sleep, for ever.' However, Danny could still reflect on what was happening to him. Intermittently he thought that he might be better off if he didn't go to hospital but tried to come to grips with his feelings. As he knew about the Crisis Centre, he asked if he could go there and still have his regular sessions with me. I agreed.

Danny stayed at the Centre for four weeks. The Centre became his chrysalis, a place where the most profound changes in his feelings and outlook could take place while he was safe and protected from all outside pressures. He has eloquently recalled his breakdown, the first days at the Centre and the dream which presaged his recovery.

The Breakdown
It didn't happen all at once, rather gradually over several weeks. My depression got worse and I couldn't cope with work, with everyday chores about the house, with even answering the phone. I was drinking very heavily and smoking a lot of pot. In the past this would help, but then it just made everything seem more negative. This culminated in the terrifying week before I went to the Centre when I became frightened of everyone around me and didn't want to go out of the house. I couldn't talk to anyone, or even to myself, I found it impossible to make any kind of reasonable explanation of the situation. I finally ended up with a complete sense of fragmentation. Literally I felt fragmented, shattered. I was a victim unable to control things, a fragment myself, whirling around. Since I was still coming to see you, I was frightened that you wouldn't believe me, that you would think it was all a ploy. It took a whole day before I could really admit to myself that I wanted to go to the Crisis Centre.

The First Days at the Centre
I arrived in the evening. I was very nervous and stayed in my room for the whole of the next day. Then I went downstairs, for breakfast I think. I met Sally and Tom. There was a very cheerful, competent atmosphere. I found it very easy to build

147

a personal relationship with Sally. I suppose I needed a woman, especially a woman with whom I wasn't having a sexual relationship, but who would be there when I felt black and gloomy, someone to talk to. I remember feeling like a derelict black, a Bowery bum, broken and beaten. In the beginning it was so bad I thought I was in Hell, then slowly, gradually the gloom began to lift. I found it would help if I could be useful, get involved in doing things like washing up, preparing food, cleaning, things like that. I also decided to do a lot of drawings, to record my dreams, my fantasies. After a couple of days another fellow came, Ritchie I think his name was, a salesman who saw monsters. I took to him right away, and I did a lot of drawings with him. He had never drawn before, but once he got started it was terrific, all sorts of images came up. We did mandalas, together and then with everyone in the house. Otherwise I spent my time going for walks in the park. When I was in the park I would just try to let everything down, immerse myself in my fantasies. Mostly they continued on the theme of degradation, being a degraded figure, and of sad, haunting, gloomy images. Then I had an extraordinary dream, different from anything I had ever dreamed before. In every way it was a turning point.

The Dream

I was looking for my parents who were lost. I went to Paris to find them, but they weren't there. Somebody said they had gone to Spain, so I took a train and went to Spain, to Barcelona. Then I got a little bus up to the Costa Brava. I found myself on top of a cliff that reached all the way down to the sea. I sat staring at the rugged rocks. It was a bleak and wild scene. Suddenly I had the feeling that I wasn't going to find my parents, that the search had reached its end. This was very painful. I decided to return to England.

Upon my return I was back on the Finchley Road (London) walking to see my friends Mike and Molly. They have always stood for my parents. They have a large family, lots of children. I often visit them and they have looked after me. When I arrived they were just on the point of going out. They said, 'Come on, let's all go out and have a drink together.' Instead of going to our usual pub, we took a different turn and found ourselves in a completely unfamiliar part of Hampstead, where I had never been before, almost like countryside.

I discovered a very old pub on a crossroads. It seemed to have been made at different times. Some parts were very old indeed, perhaps the fourteenth or fifteenth century, and other parts were garish and modern. I went into the pub. It was composed of numerous bars and small rooms and I made my way into the main room. Immediately I was struck by the fact that the people there didn't seem to belong to this world. They seemed to belong to another world and I had the strong impression that this pub was a gateway to another realm, a gateway to time travel.

In the pub there were many kinds of evil-looking characters, crooks of various descriptions who frightened me. The owner may have been a criminal himself, I wasn't sure. He kept a large lizard with a green snout on the bar. Anyway, he was quite kind to me. He told me where to find Molly and Mike. I went into the next room and there was Molly chatting away with several people who I realized were fifteenth- or sixteenth-century highwaymen, cut-throats and rogues. As she seemed to be unaware of this, I kept trying to attract her attention, to warn her that she was talking to people from another time zone who were the most dangerous possible characters. However she wouldn't take any notice. At that moment I looked for Michael. Michael had become transformed and made invisible. But I heard his voice and he informed me that he was the archangel Michael, and that he was going to act as my guide.

He personally directed me to a small flight of stone steps that led to a very old wooden door. I walked out of the pub and found myself in a square in Italy in the seventeenth century. Now all my instructions came from Michael. Almost without hearing his words I knew what I had to do, the way I had to go. I relaxed and followed his directions. The square had a round fountain in the middle and eight roads leading away from it. Michael directed me to a road running to the east which I followed. This was a road that led backwards in time, quite literally. As I walked the houses became older and older. Finally they turned into wattle and daub huts, very very primitive wattle and daub huts, like mud and sticks. These huts could have dated back to any time. Then all the dwellings vanished and the path became a narrow straight track. Suddenly it turned to the right and then passed between high grassy banks. It was now no more than a single footpath and as I walked between the grassy banks I could see nothing on either side until I came to a slight clearing. In front of me there was a large oddly shaped mound. On top of the mound there were angelic acrobats doing the most extraordinary acrobatics, completely free from the laws of gravity. They could fly around and they could do triple somersaults in the air. They could elongate their bodies and shorten them too. Quite obviously they were not human beings, not human at all. As I looked at them in amazement, the mound vanished, along with the acrobats, and I could see that the shape of the mound and the odd shape of the road had been caused by an enormous gate that had been hidden in the mound. It was beautiful, wrought iron and covered with gold gilt. A wall led up to the gate and next to it there was a small wooden door. I went up to the door, turned the handle as I felt instructed to do by the archangel Michael, and walked through the door. Immediately I found myself transported to a different realm.

I have to say that throughout my walk backwards in time colours had been changing, becoming more and more intense, vivid. Once I walked through this door the intensification of colour increased tremendously. I found myself standing on a decorative veranda. One side of the veranda was lined with people sitting in chairs. They seemed very familiar and as I looked at them I began to recognize that they were various characters out of paintings. Now the archangel, Michael, appeared again, as an angel, and introduced me to them. There were various characters out of the paintings of Hieronymus Bosch, and there was someone from a Rembrandt. Finally I was introduced to Jesus. He was very tall and arrogant. He looked like a Greek patriarch in his forties. He had a bishop's ring on his finger. I tried to shake hands with him, but he made me kneel before him and kiss the ring.

Next to Jesus there was a black man who actually looked like a friend of mine, a really wild spade named Leroy. He was the Devil. I looked closely, he had horns and was distinctly a rogue. Still he was affable and friendly and shook my hand warmly.

Beyond the veranda and on the right side of it, there arose a cliff covered with creepers. Michael told me to walk over and look closely at them. As I got nearer I noticed that the creepers were concealing a small door. I pushed them aside and saw the word H E L L, written in iron letters. I tried the door, but it was locked. Then Michael handed me a rather ornate heavy black iron key which fitted perfectly inside the lock. I turned the key, opened the door and looked inside. Inside there was an enormously deep pit which widened at the centre. I looked up at the roof. There was a mandala made up of the elements of an electric grill. It was glowing red hot and made the most beautiful pattern. A terrific heat emanated from the roof as well as from the depths of the pit. Wisps of smoke also arose from the pit and from rocks along its sides. On these rocks lizards and various demonic creatures sat glowing against the flames below.

I knew I had the choice of entering the pit or simply closing the door. I felt that I was unable to enter the pit. So I closed the door and as I did so, the nature of this place occurred to me. I realized that it was a zone between the living and the dead, and that the spirits of the dead could visit the living in this place. I also realized that the search for my parents was continuing, and, in fact, that the search was specifically for my mother. Although she was dead, I had been directed to this place in order to meet her.

At that moment a figure appeared dressed in a black cloak which ran down to its feet. It stood at an angle to me with a cowl hiding its face. As soon as I became aware of it, the figure started to walk across a grassy plain that led out of the veranda. I hesitated but Michael instructed me to follow it. Then he said, 'I shall be leaving you now.'

The figure was like an hallucination. One instant it would be there, then it would seem to vanish. I followed it over gently rolling countryside, no trees, just endlessly rolling grassy plains. The horizon was at least twenty miles distant, yet every single blade of grass was in clear focus, no matter how far away it was. The light was intense and the grass continued to be in clear focus for mile after mile. I followed the figure in a completely timeless way for what could have been hours or days. I felt relaxed and happy, as intended. I was not impatient. After a while I realized that I had been gradually climbing. Although I was on a gently rolling plain, I had been making a slow ascent. Finally I reached the highest place on this whole plain. The horizon now stretched almost infinitely far on all sides. I was on the top of a hill. Near me there was a flat rock on which the figure had lain down, arms outstretched, face upwards, but still hidden by the cowl. It seemed to be beckoning me. I felt that I had to go and lie on the figure face down with my palms touching its palms. It was as if I were about to be crucified.

I went and lay down upon it. As I did I became aware that the figure was my mother. Then this image of my mother began to undergo many kaleidoscopic transformations. Each was familiar and important to me, as if all my relatives, both alive and dead, were flickering through this figure. Suddenly the figure became solid and substantial, and I realized that the person I was lying on was you. I had a terrific feeling of relief and support. All my cares and worries seemed to blow away, all my anxieties ceased. I seemed to lose consciousness and then I woke up.

The Recovery

Upon awakening I felt clear and refreshed as well as immensely reassured. I realized that the Crisis Centre was truly a secure and comforting place. Within a short time I made plans to visit my home and begin sorting out the mess I had left behind. I became much more active at the Centre, helping with the cooking and cleaning and generally taking a keen interest in everything going on. I also resumed my teaching schedule with a degree of enthusiasm I had not experienced for a long while. While my depression and anxiety did not altogether leave me, they returned to normal, that is tolerable levels. I left the Centre two weeks later without the feeling of dread which had hung over me for so long. I could look forward to the future.

Danny's transformation followed in the tradition of John Perceval, John (the Butterfly Man) and the many others who have demonstrated a renewed relationship with themselves and others by a dream, vision or reverie. With Danny the passage from psychic fragmentation to emotional reconstruction was made possible by his unconscious acceptance of the help that Sally, Tom and myself could give him. He recognized that we could guide him through the rocks and reefs of his hostility and hatred without our being injured or destroyed and without our leaving him as had his mother, wife and girlfriend. He established us as a solid, substantial presence within himself, and, in so doing, reestablished his belief that reality could be benevolent and it was safe to be sane.

Subsequently, Danny has continued the work begun in his therapy and as revealed in the dramatic events at the Crisis Centre. He still gets depressed, but not nearly so severely. He still gets anxious, but he is not incapacitated by it. Generally his life has taken a turn for the better.

*

In the four-year period, January 1973 through February 1977, we have answered hundreds of inquiries and requests for assistance. These were made by people in all walks of life and from many parts of the British Isles, as well as Europe and America.

Acute depression was the most common situation in which we were asked to intervene. Other crises included acute psychoses, recurrent psychoses, manic states and a variety of problems which can be assumed under the categories of family and adolescent crises and anti-social behaviour. Most crises involved two to four people although not all necessarily stayed at the centre at once. The average duration of intervention was two weeks, although some were as short as one day and others lasted for several months.

The most frequent outcome of a crisis, as it abated or was resolved, was for all concerned to go home and carry on with their lives. Where this was impractical, or further support was needed, guests moved to other Arbours communities or stayed with friends or relatives. Anyone who has stayed at the centre knows that he is welcome to drop in any time and to attend the monthly meetings of the Arbours communities.[11]

Significantly, we do not use and have not had to use either tranquillizing or anti-depressive medications as an adjunct to our crisis work. To the best of my knowledge the Arbours Crisis Centre is unique in this respect.[12] During these four years, and subsequently, it has been satisfying to provide a place where people could benefit from a period of depression, regression or psychosis. As a young married woman stated, some months after being at the centre, it was indeed 'an alternative sanctuary from which I was able, in time, to emerge to find my dignity and my nervous system intact and my potential unprejudiced'.[13]

It has also been satisfying to point out to people that they did not have to 'go mad' in order to work through a crisis situation. This happened with 'Sylvia', a middle-aged schoolteacher who felt about to explode after juggling a home, a career, marriage and children for years. Before she left the centre, she wrote an open letter,

To anyone who comes here:

I came here to be among mad people like myself. I imagined a house of chaos and complete disintegration of the mind. I could smell the place. I thought there would be shit and pee everywhere, that music of all types would be sounding throughout the place. I was afraid to wear my engagement ring for fear of it being stolen while I slept ... But the house looked clean and comfortable. It had an aura of tranquillity. Everything seemed to fall into shape without effort. I felt nothing was expected of me ...

I talked a lot to Sally and Tom. They are great listeners. Sometimes they explain things that make sense ... As I write, Sally is upstairs, cleaning, but I know she will come if I want her. Tom has had to go out but he promised not to be too long. I have laughed and cried a lot with Sally and Tom. They laugh with me but they don't cry ...

I haven't had to go mad here.

Notes

1. Erich Lindemann, 'Symptomology and management of acute grief', *American Journal of Psychiatry*, 101 (September 1944).

2. Gerald Caplan, *Principles of Preventive Psychiatry* (New York, Basic Books, 1964), pp. 40–41.

3. There is an extensive but diffuse literature concerning crisis intervention. The following anthologies and review papers are good references and provide further access to the literature.

Howard J. Parad, *Crisis Intervention: Selected Reading* (New

I Haven't Had to Go Mad Here

York, Family Service Association of America, 1965); Allen Darbonne, 'Crisis: a review of theory, practice and research', *Psychotherapy: Theory, Research and Practice*, 4, no. 2 (May 1967), pp. 371–9; Katharine Eastham *et al.*, 'The concept of crisis', *Canadian Psychiatric Association Journal*, 15 (1970), pp. 463–72; W. Claiborn and G. Specter, *Crisis Intervention* (New York, Behavioural Publications, 1973); Donna Aguilera and Janice Messick, *Crisis Intervention: Theory and Methodology* (St Louis, C. V. Mosby, 1974); Donald Langsley *et al.*, *The Treatment of Families in Crisis* (New York, Grune and Stratton, 1968); Colin Murray Parkes, *Bereavement: Studies of Grief in Adult Life* (London, Penguin, 1972).

4. Donald Langsley *et al.*, *The Treatment of Families in Crisis*; Donald Langsley *et al.*, 'Family crisis therapy: results and implications', *Family Process*, 7, no. 2 (September 1968), pp. 145–58.

5. K. Flomenhaft, D. Langsley and P. Machotka, 'Follow-up evaluation of family crisis therapy', *American Journal of Orthopsychiatry*, 39, no. 5 (October 1969), pp. 753–9; K. Flomenhaft, D. Langsley and P. Machotka, 'Avoiding mental hospital admission: a follow-up study' *American Journal of Psychiatry*, 127, no. 10 (April 1971), pp. 127–30.

6. R. D. Scott, 'Cultural frontiers in the mental health service', *Schizophrenic Bulletin*, no. 10 (Fall 1974), pp. 58–73.

7. David Smith, 'Historical perspectives on the national free clinic movement', *Free Medical Clinics: Innovations in Health Care Delivery*, ed. J. Scharz (US Government Printing Office, Washington, D C; Caroline Coon and Rufus Harris, *The Release Report on Drug Offenders and the Law* (London, Sphere Books, 1969); James Gorden, 'Coming together: consultation with young people', *Social Policy* (July–August 1974), pp. 40–52; Heavy Daze formerly *Copeman*, magazine of the Cope Trust, 15 Acklam Road, London W10).

8. Chad Varah (ed.), *Samaritans in the 70s* (London, Constable, 1973). There are also branches of the Samaritans in India, Australia, Hong Kong, Singapore and Brazil.

9. From 1953 to 1973 the suicide rate in England has dropped from 11.5 suicides per 100,000 year, to 8 suicides per 100,000.

10. Tom Ryan and Sally Berry were the resident therapists at the Arbours Crisis Centre from 1973 to 1975.

Andrea Sabbadini and Laura Forti were the resident therapists from 1975 to 1977. Now they, too, serve as team leaders.

From autumn 1977 to summer 1978 the resident therapists were David Rose and Diana de Vigili. Since summer 1978 the resident therapists have been Bob and Iona Grant.

11. See the Appendix for a detailed consideration of interventions involving a stay at the crisis centre related to sex, age, marriage status, occupation, nationality, length of stay, reason for intervention, and outcome.

12. A small percentage of people have come to the Arbours Centre heavily tranquillized. We have found that these people do better if they diminish or eliminate this medication, no matter what their presenting difficulties. Not infrequently medication and over-medication contribute to the very crisis from which a person is trying to disentangle himself or herself.

The American psychiatrist, Maurice Rappaport, formerly chief researcher at Agnews State Hospital in California, has reported, for example, that young people going through their first or second psychotic experience do better if they do *not* receive medication when treated at hospital. Patients who were off drugs in the hospital and stayed off after they left were less likely to return to hospital. They showed greater adjustment in the community, greater autonomy, more ability to get along with others, and better skill at providing for the necessities of life. Dr Rappaport demonstrated that patients who benefited most from not being drugged were those who had been well adjusted prior to the onset of their psychosis and who showed paranoid symptoms at admission. He suggests that medication interferes with efforts by these people to work through their problems. The psychotic symptoms may actually reflect a healthy struggle to come to terms with personal or interpersonal difficulties (*Behaviour Today*, 6, no. 35 (30 September 1974), pp. 252–3).

13. Joy Melville, 'Helping people to survive a crisis', *New Society*, 46, no. 836 (12 October 1978), pp. 78–9.

7 The Green Hand

I was driving north on the motorway. I'm a salesman, you
know, anything that comes my way, rugs, furniture, lamps, odd
lots. Anyway, just as I was approaching Manchester, this thing
appeared on the bonnet. It was green, as big as a man. It reminded me of some creature from outer space. I slammed on
the brakes and got out of the car but it had disappeared. I was
really scared. So I got off the motorway. I have a friend in
Manchester and I decided to head there and catch a rest at her
place. Then, no sooner had I calmed down, than it came back
again. But this time it didn't go away and it started to pound
on the bonnet. Again I stopped the car and got out to investigate. Took a hammer with me too. The creature just sat on the
bonnet and refused to get off. I screamed at it. Nothing happened. I screamed some more. Then it slid off and came at me.
I thought it would do me, but I was able to knock it to the
ground and bash it on the head. It fell over and didn't move.
It was dead. I started to shake. Then I noticed a police station
down the road. I ran over and pulled at the sergeant. 'Come
quickly, someone's attacked me and I think I've killed him.'
The whole station poured out and ran with me to the car.
Imagine my surprise when I discovered the creature wasn't
there. Then I realized why. He had been a Martian. As soon as
I had run away his friends must have come and got him. Anyway no one believed me. They were very angry. They forced
me to go back to the station. Later I was taken to a place and
given a shot. It put me to sleep. I awoke in the nuthouse. I
knew it was the nuthouse. I had been there before, a couple of

159

years back, after I had tried to kill myself. The same faces, the same smells.

Then the green thing came again, appeared at the window. Only this time it was only its hand, a green hand. I screamed and lunged for the hand. It disappeared. But I cut myself on the window as it shattered. They asked me what had happened. I wasn't going to lie to them. I pleaded for them to save me from this second creature. I was sure it was another one trying to get even for what I had done to the one on the bonnet. No one believed me. They just gave me another shot. The next day it came back again. I can't remember what happened next. My mind's all hazy. But I'm told I broke every window in the place. Eventually it stopped coming. I was so doped up I could hardly think. Two months later they let me out. They asked me if I saw anything. I said no but I didn't mention I was still scared the creature would come back. I couldn't eat. I couldn't sleep. Then my sister told me about this place, Harbours she called it, where they help people like me. I didn't want to go. I thought it was another nuthouse. But she insisted. So we went to this house. It smelled good; someone had just made a chocolate cake. The people all looked alike. I couldn't figure out who was supposed to help me. Then this fellow came over, big with a black beard. I didn't know he was the shrink. Everyone called him Joe. He asked me what had happened. I told him the whole story. Why not? I hoped he would give me a shot and put me to sleep. But he didn't, he just listened, carefully. And he didn't fidget like the others had done at the hospital. Then he said he understood what had happened to me. He knew all about the green creatures. He was an expert in green creatures. He said I should not worry because they rarely came to this house. But if they did, do nothing, but call him right away. He would come over and help me fight them. He also said that the others in the house knew about creatures too. Just talk to them whenever I was frightened. I didn't think that would help. But the funny thing is, the creatures didn't come back. And then another fellow came by. He was an artist-type. Did all sorts of drawings with me. You know, I never drew before. But he got me to draw the creatures, and I felt better. Eventually I learned that the creatures were part of me, or something. That took a while. But the house was good. I stayed there three weeks. No shots or nothing. Then I went back north to see my girl.

This account, reconstructed from several conversations with a man who stayed at the Arbours Crisis Centre, illustrates the two basic principles of crisis care: calm in the face of another person's anxiety, and respect for what another person is thinking or feeling even though it may seem unusual, strange or extraordinary.

We endeavour to practise these principles at the communities of the Arbours Association. Dr Leon Redler and his colleagues try to do likewise at the houses they have established in London as do the Soteria house communities which have been established in the United States by Dr Loren Mosher, Alma Menn and Leonard Goveia.

Many other groups have endeavoured to provide comparable support. But their ability to do so is hampered by an adherence to physical treatments or by a lack of expertise. Others are restricted because the care of distressed individuals is not their primary function: 'hippie' communes tend to be quite tolerant of bizarre behaviour and personal disturbance and accept as members or guests young people who might otherwise wind up in mental hospital. Many of these households have assumed the function of therapeutic communities, the more serious of them providing sanctuary and hospitality in a manner not unlike the East London community, Kingsley Hall.[1]

Kingsley Hall was a centre of social innovation for five years. The community dispersed in 1970 because the lease on the building could not be renewed. Thereafter, the

Arbours Association was founded. Concomitantly Dr Leon Redler, an American psychiatrist who had lived at Kingsley Hall and was still involved with the community, decided to find alternative accommodation for some of the residents.[2] After many difficulties he rented several buildings in the Archway area of North London which were scheduled for demolition by the local council.

The new houses were decrepit, uncomfortable and lacking in basic amenities. Windows were broken, walls were cracked and damp oozed through the floors and broken plasterboard. They seemed to mirror the despair, hopelessness and insecurity of the people who began to inhabit them. But they also reflected the potential for change and reconstruction which Leon saw as an essential feature of an emotional breakdown.

These houses became known as the Archway community.[3] On leaving, one young man said,

I came here because I believed I had lost my voice, my self, my reason. I found none of these 'things' and now no longer expect to, or even want to. What I discovered instead was a place where I could at last be lost enough to say so ...[4]

William Saunders lived in the Archway community for a year and a half.[5] His role carried with it no formal title, although 'social therapist' might do justice to a few of his responsibilities. Will prefers the term 'facilitator' because he was constantly engaged in facilitating the existence of the community. He made sure that utilities were connected and working and that basic repairs were done. This task was continuous because the houses were old and many residents looked upon them as an embodiment of a despised parent or a hated aspect of themselves. The kitchen was the particular object of ambivalence. Once cleaned or painted it was soon defaced. Food was left about to rot, yoghurt grew spontaneously from cartons. In disgust Will once carried out nearly a hundred empty milk bottles that had been piling up.

Yet the terrible conditions of the houses and their subsequent mistreatment was part of the ethos of the community and was seen as an advantage. It symbolized a tacit decision by the group to allow its psychotic members to express their despair and murderous antagonisms, rather than bottle them in. It was better to break windows than remain catatonic or contained by tranquillizers. That the houses were in a run-down neighbourhood also helped because there were few adjacent families to be bothered by screams and cries. For all the anger in the air, most of the violence remained silently unexpressed. When it did become overt, the houses and furnishing bore the brunt of the damage. Attacks by one person against another were not tolerated. Two rules were clear cut: don't murder another resident, and pay your rent. As for creature comforts, those who missed them simply left.

Will's most important task was to be around and available for people to talk to when they wanted to do so. He did not 'give therapy', nor did he interpret to other residents what he thought they were doing in fantasy (for this many had individual therapists from outside the household). Leon Redler visited weekly for a group meeting at which both personal and communal problems could be discussed. Leon also came when the community wanted assistance in dealing with a disturbance it could not contain. The community preferred this arrangement and did not want therapists or designated 'helpers' to live in.

Help was given, but it was rarely defined as help, and it was never imposed. It just seemed to materialize because people were available to be with when they were distressed. Leon, Will and other residents went to great lengths to ensure that people were accepted on their own terms and not invalidated because of bizarre or socially inappropriate behaviour. Often this meant staying up all night with guests like the frenzied lady who was 'trying to find something that's been lost'. Leon took trouble to ensure that there were fresh flowers in her room because she had previously mentioned that she liked flowers. He knew that her room would soon be in a shambles and the flowers strewn about but hoped that at some level of awareness she would appreciate the gesture and therefore choose to make contact with him.

Similar efforts were made on behalf of Eric, a thirty-year-old man who came to the community after many years in many mental hospitals. The household referred to him as 'the dead one' because he rarely spoke and had been in a catatonic state for over fifteen years. In three years he gradually 'came alive' with the assistance and forbearance of the whole community and especially Haya Oakley, an Israeli therapist who spent most time with him.

Coming alive involved tremendous outbursts of aggression towards the houses and everyone in them. Three times he practically wrecked the place, throwing furniture out of the windows and breaking everything around him. At one point the only thing Haya could do was to wrap him in a blanket and sit on him until he calmed down.

Yet his anger represented a tremendous advance. Withdrawn, head stooped, he had refused to talk with anyone except his mother, and even with her only on certain occasions. Finding out what he needed or wanted had presented great difficulty, and only after he had been in the community a long while were people able to communicate with him. Will discovered that although he would not talk, he would write. So notes were written between him and Will and others. Eventually he went shopping by himself and would give a note to the shopkeeper of the food he wanted.

Will recalls the moment when the usual barriers that separated Eric and him seemed to part. It was late at night. Will was about to settle down with a brandy, as was his custom after a hard day. Then there was a loud knock on the door.

'Come in.'

Slowly the door creaked open. Eric appeared.

'Come in.'

Eric remained half in and half out.

'Do you want to talk?'

'Nooooooooooooooo.'

'Would you like to sit down.'

'Yeeeeeeeeeeeessssssss.'

'I was about to have a brandy and a cigar. Would you like some?'

'Yesssssssssss.'

So Eric came in, sat down on a chair, sipped the brandy and smoked the cigar. An hour went by. Will felt very tired. He told Eric how he felt and said he wanted to go to sleep. Would he leave and come another evening?

Eric said, 'Yesssssssssss,' and ambled back to his room. But their relationship was on a new footing.

Since this incident, the community itself has greatly changed. The original houses have been demolished by the council and people have moved to other houses in the general vicinity. But the work continues, now in association with the Philadelphia Association.[6] Altogether there are seven households, some in new houses with gardens, and one has a pottery and glasshouse.

Soteria House is the third project to be stimulated by the

theory and practice of the Kingsley Hall community. It is the brainchild of Dr Loren Mosher, of the Center for Studies of Schizophrenia, National Institute of Mental Health in Rockville, Maryland, and his colleagues.[7] Loren had long been impressed by the psycho-social and non-somatic (absence of drugs or electroshock) treatment of acutely disturbed individuals. However, he was also keenly aware of the lack of firm evidence as to the effectiveness of this work. After several visits to Kingsley Hall, and the Arbours and Archway communities, he became determined to pioneer a kindred effort in the United States. Moreover, he decided that this work would be most useful if it could also serve as a research vehicle in order to provide objective data as to the value of interpersonal interventions in crisis situations and with people who would be diagnosed as schizophrenic.

Soteria – from the Greek word for deliverance – started in 1971 in a large, comfortable, communally run house in San Jose, California.[8] The residents include two staff and up to six patients. The staff work three days on and three days off and are assisted and supervised by the project director, Ms Alma Menn (who previously worked on an experimental ward of Agnews State Hospital; the entire project bears the stamp of her previous experience and strong personal presence). Greater emphasis is placed on the definition of staff and patients than at the Arbours or Archway communities. However, as the staff and patients often look alike, dress alike and perform similar chores, the casual visitor might have great difficulty in distinguishing one from the other.

The staff are non-professionals who have been chosen for their ability to tune in to the tortured and bizarre or dreamlike states of reality which the patients inhabit, and they are expected to serve as guides, reassuring, supporting and protecting the people they are with.

At Soteria House a psychosis is not viewed as a disease or part of an inexorable process of personal and emotional disintegration. It is seen as an altered state of consciousness that has occurred because of an intense intra- or interpersonal crisis. This crisis, the psychosis and any attendant regression, present an opportunity for learning, growth and the development of a stronger and more integrated personality and identity, and some patients are allowed to go through their psychosis instead of having it altered or terminated by tranquillizing drugs. A brief quote from the Soteria brochure illustrates this point of view:

It is believed that by allowing and helping the resident to gradually work with and through this crisis in living, or schizophrenia, he will be better able to understand himself and his fears. So rather than ignoring or quelling this altered state, he will explore it, understand it, and finally learn from it.

It is noteworthy that the staff does not give individual psychotherapy, nor are the residents encouraged to have sessions with outside therapists. But they can and do spend long hours talking with others about the nature of their experiences. These sessions are patently therapeutic in that people find that their experiences are worth while, and that they are given the emotional space to get on with their 'trip'.[9]

Although formal meetings at the house are few, there are many impromptu meetings when staff members spend time with residents who are especially distressed. There are no time limits to these sessions, which may last many hours, or even days. This was the case with Marjorie, a young college student who came to the house after her roommates found her trying to electrocute herself. She believed she was the devil and that the T V was giving her messages to 'burn, baby, burn, feel the fire of hell'. The girl felt she was so bad, she had to die. One morning, a week after her arrival, she set fire to her mattress and clothes. Fortunately the residents smelled the smoke and put out the fire. Marjorie was not hurt and after she had put on some new clothes, a number of residents took her to the dining room and began to explore exactly what had happened. At first she remained like a zombie. But after a while and with some encouragement she described recent events in her family including the death and cremation of her grandfather, with whom she had been very close (and wanted to join), and a bitter sexual rivalry with her elder sister whom she wished would die.

Many hours later Marjorie began to come together. Instead of maintaining a blank face, she cried at the thought of her grandfather, became angry at the mention of her sister and was appropriately depressed while conveying details of her disastrous sex life. Most importantly, she began to appreciate that there were connections between her bizarre attempts at suicide, her preoccupation with the devil, and her relationship to her grandmother and sister. No one interpreted these issues to her. She realized them herself, over an entire day, and in the continual presence of one young man. He was a staff member who by staying with her and by not becoming impatient, frightened or critical of what she said or did, was able to demonstrate to Marjorie that her feelings were real, comprehensible and tolerable.

Regrettably there exist few other places where a person like Marjorie would be allowed the time, space and encouragement to find out about herself and in her own way. In 1961 Drs Albert Honig and Harold Fine founded the Delaware

Valley Mental Health Foundation, a service, training and research centre in Pennsylvania.[10] There a unique form of residential analytic 'family therapy' is practised. Two to five severely disturbed individuals live in a small, comfortable house together with a professional couple who provide intensive physical care, emotional support, a warm family atmosphere and psychotherapy according to their degree of expertise.[11] There are several such houses set amid fourteen acres of rolling hills, the remnants of two early American farms.

Number Nine and Diabasis are two other projects of exceptional interest. Number Nine was a crisis centre located in downtown New Haven, Connecticut, started in 1969 by Dennis and Yvonne Jaffe and Ted Clark and kept going until 1974. Housed in a couple of derelict buildings which they fixed up, the centre intervened in many situations including drug overdoses and runaway children. Young people who had 'flipped out' stayed there, received sympathetic care and were able to avoid overzealous psychiatric treatment.[12]

In 1973 the Jungian psychoanalyst, Dr John Weir Perry, and his colleagues opened a house in San Francisco where young people could go through a first psychotic episode without heavy medication, shock therapy or pervasive social restrictions. Called Diabasis after the Greek word meaning 'crossing-over', the centre initially took six guests on a day-care basis. Later this was extended to full-time residence.[13]

Dr Perry believes, as do the Soteria and London groups, that a psychosis can set the stage for 'profound recollections' whereby a person can 'get in touch with an otherwise lost vision of the meaning of things'. Thus, a psychosis is not an illness but an inner journey which crosses into ultimately important psychological and spiritual realms.[14] Diabasis was meant to be a refuge where people who have been going through this journey could understand it and discover its healing potential.

Group homes and half-way houses are less dramatic alternatives to institutionalization and have become increasingly popular since the 1960s. Some are quite strict and insist that residents leave the house during the day and take heavy doses of tranquillizers. Others allow the residents a great deal of autonomy and are run as an admixture of therapeutic community and hippie commune. They extend support, care and after-care to a large variety of people including those who have been diagnosed as neurotic, psychotic and plain bad (the so-called sociopath). Where the community has been set up to rehabilitate alcoholics or drug addicts the use of any psycho-active agents is generally forbidden.

The Richmond Fellowship, in particular, has been successful in providing facilities for individuals and families who have been under severe emotional strain. The Fellowship is a private mental health charity and is directed by Ms Elly Jansen. Elly came to London from Holland in 1959 to study theology and took a degree in divinity. During her studies she rented a spacious house in Richmond, Surrey and invited patients who had been discharged from a local mental hospital to share the house with her. The impetus to do so came from her previous experience loking after autistic and emotionally disturbed children (when she found that peers can be of great help to one another). Moreover, her religious beliefs led her to conclude that formal religion 'was too concerned with teaching people dogma and too little with teaching people about people'.[15]

Elly endured the first months in her new home without financial, professional or moral support. She was a student in a foreign land and under constant harassment from local authorities for contravening rarely enforced building regulations. She was also harassed for working without a permit, although she received no salary and lived as an equal in the community. She carried on, aided by the enthusiasm of others who eventually joined her and by their willingness to learn from each other, with the firm conviction that it was possible to make contact with even the most disturbed person.

Being more unaware than most people of what constitutes 'normal behaviour', my very innocence stood me in good stead. It allowed me to understand eccentric behaviour partly because I expected little in the way of conformity; at the same time it led me to have expectations in terms of talents, mutual concern, and fulfilling obligations because I had no reason not to have them.[16]

Since 1959 Elly and her co-workers have established a network of thirty-five half-way houses in Britain, Australia and the United States. These provide residential and day care for hundreds of people each year. They have helped to eliminate many a 'revolving door' situation whereby someone is sent to hospital, treated, sent back to the very environment which contributed to the breakdown in the first place, and then winds up in hospital again. The Richmond Fellowship also runs extensive training programmes in human relations and group work, and assists other groups wanting to start half-way houses.[17]

The achievements of Elly and the Richmond Fellowship, as well as those of the other groups that I have been describing, point out what individuals and local organizations can accomplish when the emphasis of psychiatric intervention changes from social control to communication and sympathetic containment.

Notes

1. For further information about the Kingsley Hall community, see Mary Barnes and Joseph Berke, *Mary Barnes: Two Accounts of a Journey through Madness* (London, Hart-Davis MacGibbon, 1971); Morton Schatzman, 'Madness and morals', *The Radical Therapist* (New York, Ballantine Books, 1971), pp. 65–96; Oliver Gillie, 'Freedom Hall', *New Society*, no. 339 (27 March 1969), pp. 473–5; James Gordon, 'Who is mad? Who is sane?'; R. D. Laing: 'In search of a new psychiatry', *Going Crazy*, ed. H. R. Ruitenbeck (New York, Bantam Books, 1972), pp. 65–102.

2. Leon Redler was assisted by Mike Yocum and Paul Zeal.

3. *Asylum* is a documentary film made about one of the households in the Archway Community, produced and directed by Peter Robinson and Associates, USA, 1971.

4. Vin and Pat Rosenthal, 'With Leon (and Laing) in London: an interview with Leon Redler', *Voices* (Winter 1973/4), p. 49.

5. William Saunders is an American who came to London to further his studies as a graduate in human relations. He has lived and worked in London with Arbours Association and as a psychotherapist.

6. The present members of the Philadelphia Association include Francis Huxley, R. D. Laing, Leon Redler, Hugh Crawford and J. M. Heaton. The mailing address is: 74a Portland Road, London W11.

7. My discussion about Soteria House is based on several meetings with Dr Loren Mosher and Ms Alma Menn and also the following: Alma Menn, 'Growing at Soteria', *In Search of Therapy*, ed. Dennis Jaffe (New York, Harper Colophon Books, 1975), pp. 84–99; L. Goveia, A. Menn and L. Mosher, 'Schizophrenia and Crisis Therapy' (paper presented at the Annual Meeting of the American Orthopsychiatry Association, Detroit, Michigan, April 1972); A. Menn, L. Mosher and A. Reifman, 'Characteristics of nonprofessionals serving as

primary therapists for acute schizophrenics', *Hospital and Community Psychiatry*, 24, no. 6 (6 June 1973), pp. 391–6; A. Menn, L. Mosher and A. Reifman, 'A new treatment for schizophrenia: does it work?', ibid. (April 1973).

8. For further information about Soteria contact Mental Research Institute, 555 Middlefield Road, Palo Alto, California. Since 1975 a second Soteria house has been established in San Mateo, California.

9. Results of follow-up studies indicate that the project's unhurried, self-healing approach is as effective as the standard régime of brief hospitalization and phenothiazine treatment. Significantly, people who attended the Soteria programme showed a marked increase in psycho-social functioning as compared with those who did not. A. Menn, L. Mosher and S. Matthews, 'Soteria: evaluation of a home-based treatment for schizophrenia', *American Journal of Orthopsychiatry*, 43, no. 3 (April 1975), pp. 455–67.

10. Delaware Valley Mental Health Foundation, 833 East Butler Avenue, Doylestown, Pennsylvania.

11. Albert Honig, *The Awakening Nightmare: A Breakthrough in Treating the Mentally Ill* (Rockaway, N.J., The American Faculty Press, 1972). See also *Other Voices*, a documentary film about the work of Dr Honig available from Delaware Valley Mental Health Foundation.

12. Dennis Jaffe, 'Creating a counter-institution', *The Radical Therapist*, ed. J. Agel (New York, Ballantine Books, 1971), pp. 219–34; Dennis Jaffe, 'The healer, the community, or the bureaucrat', *In Search of Therapy*, pp. 47–60; D. and Y. Jaffe, 'Sara's odyssey: acid and the youth culture', *Going Crazy*, ed. H. Ruitenbeck, pp. 277–300; H. Ruitenbeck (ed.), 'Change within a counter-cultural crisis intervention centre', *Going Crazy*, pp. 209–32.

13. Allen Krebs, 'Some alternatives to psychiatric hospitals in the Bay area', *Arbours Network*, no. 7 (Fall 1974), p. 24.

14. John Weir Perry, *The Far Side of Madness* (New Jersey, Spectrum, 1974), pp. 5–6.

15. Oliver Gillie, 'Richmond Fellows', *New Society* (1 January 1970), p. 5.

16. Elly Jansen, 'The role of the halfway house in community mental health programs in the United Kingdom and America', *American Journal of Psychiatry*, 126, no. 10 (April 1970), p. 1500.

17. The Richmond Fellowship Annual Reports are obtainable from the Richmond Fellowship, 8 Addison Road, London W14.

8 Families by Choice

Haverville is a pleasant tree-lined suburb of Philadelphia. Large modern houses stand amid acres of grass while neighbours are not separated by fences. After the men have left for their offices in the morning, the wives easily pass from house to house for morning coffee. Later, after school, the children tear across the lawns with their dogs, cats and other assorted pets.

Dave and Joan Parnell lived in Haverville for several years before the course of their lives was suddenly altered. He was thirty-three years old, tall, thin and well established as a junior partner in a law firm. She was thirty-one, also tall, red-haired and seemingly cheerful. Before getting married, Joan had worked as an elementary school teacher. Since having twin sons five years previously, she had stayed at home and kept occupied looking after the boys, her husband and a sheepdog named Rusty.

Beneath their social veneer, neither Dave nor Joan were especially happy. They liked each other, but Dave kept worrying about business and working long hours at the office. His wife had periods of nervous depression soothed over by various multicoloured pills. Both had attended the odd encounter group, but found them more provocative than helpful. Their favoured means of relaxation was meeting with friends for drinks and a meal once the children had been put to bed.

I Haven't Had to Go Mad Here

Joan began to suffer from headaches the day after her children, Chris and Sam, started to attend school. She complained and took more pills for the headaches, but they continued, and she seemed to get more irritable at home. Nothing satisfied her, yet she was not satisfied with doing nothing. She tried some part-time teaching, but found the trip into town too taxing. She tried to make some clothes for the boys, but gave that up too, because she couldn't concentrate.

Easter passed. Joan began to withdraw into herself so slowly that her husband hardly noticed. When weekends came around and he had to make the Sunday dinner, he didn't mind because he liked to cook. What disturbed him was that there was never any food in the house so he had to spend most of Sunday morning doing the shopping as well.

The flash point came very suddenly. One day Dave got a call at the office from a neighbour and friend, Mark Gross. He had returned home for lunch and found Joan wandering through his house. When he asked her what was the matter, she screamed and ran out, taking with her a few objects from the kitchen and a bottle of milk. Then the boys had stopped by. They were hungry and upset. There had been no lunch for them. Worse, Joan had locked herself in her bedroom and refused to come out.

When Dave arrived home, he found a bevy of friends and neighbours in the house. One couple was making dinner. Another was about to take his boys out to the movies. Others were trying to get Joan to come out of the bedroom. It turned out that his house had been run by his friends for a week and he hadn't noticed. In fact, he knew something was wrong, but whenever he asked his wife, she would mutter, 'It's okay, okay', and it wasn't in his nature to pursue things any further. When problems arose, he preferred to forget them.

The front doorbell rang. Another neighbour came in. She was very angry. Joan had twice walked into her house, taken a pack of cigarettes and walked out. She yelled that Joan should be put away. She knew all about these things. Joan was crazy. Her husband, a psychologist, agreed. He said Joan was psychotic and should be sent to hospital. What she needed was a long rest and drugs. Otherwise Joan was a menace. The neighbourhood couldn't have mad people running about. Her children were frightened. Her cat was frightened. It was making her sick. If something wasn't done promptly, she would call the police.

With that, the bedroom door opened and Joan walked out. She was naked except for a sheet wrapped loosely around her body.

'Please, please,' she whispered. 'Don't send me to hospital. I don't want to go to hospital. I would kill myself first. I will be all right. Please, everyone, go home and leave me alone.'

Dave didn't know what to do. On one side there was Joan begging to be left alone. On the other there was the lady from across the street yelling for a doctor.

Mark came to the rescue. Quietly he asked everyone to calm down. He passed around a bottle of brandy and arranged for coffee and sandwiches to be made. Then he thanked the distraught neighbour for letting everyone know about her concerns. Yes, there were problems, but he didn't think that Joan was a menace. If Joan bothered her again, she should feel free to call him at any time. Otherwise everything would be taken care of. Reassured, the woman went home.

Next Mark turned to Joan. Gently, he suggested that she

177

might be better off in hospital. There she would get plenty of care and would have time to get things together. Again Joan refused. He paused for a cigarette. Other people sipped their coffee. Dave buried his head in his hands.

Finally Mark made another suggestion. He reminded everyone that he was a social worker and had a lot of experience with distressed families. At his clinic he and his colleagues had been trying a new approach to crisis situations. Instead of putting people suffering from a nervous breakdown in hospital, they would help them to remain with their families. They did this by arranging a wide network of support for everyone in the family. After all, when one person was distressed, everyone else was usually involved. Moreover, Mark noted that hospitalization could make matters worse by transforming the breakdown of an individual into a family breakdown. Perhaps, if everyone was willing, this new approach could be tried with Joan and her family. It would mean a lot of work, and a lot of people would have to take part. But it might keep Joan out of hospital and help her through her emotional crisis. It might also keep the family together.

Joan whispered something incoherently and returned to bed. Dave didn't know if anything would help, but he would give it a try. Other people were enthusiastic. It was decided to arrange a meeting the following evening of everyone who might be willing to help. In the meanwhile, Mark said he would stay for the night, and a couple of other friends offered to make dinner and take the children to school in the morning.

On the day of the meeting Joan wavered between an anxious concern that the boys get to school on time and an aggressive withdrawal from those about her. For long periods she would sit curled up in bed. Then, suddenly, she would leap up, prance about, and hurl venom at whoever was in her path. Always an articulate woman but forever shy, Joan began to let fly thirty-odd years of suppressed anger and rage. It was not an easy task. She was frightened by her words and would frequently lapse into anguished sobs accompanied by violent shakes and shivers.

Dave awoke depressed and resentful towards his wife and friends for making his life so difficult. Deep down he was eager to leave the house and go to work, but he pretended to want to stay home and look after things. Only after he had screamed at the boys for wetting their beds and accidentally broken a bottle of milk did he follow Mark's advice to 'cool it' and let others help with the housework. Seeing that the children were being cared for and sensing his aggravation with Joan, he retreated to his office for the duration of the afternoon.

Amid all the turmoil, Mark remained calm but busy. He had stayed up most of the night talking with Dave and soothing Joan. He had not been put off by her verbal abuse. If anything, he was amused by her sarcasm and fascinated by her incisive comments about family, friends and neighbours. These were the very people whom he was trying to get to the helpers' meeting. Given what Joan was saying about them, he never imagined how successful his organizational efforts would be.

Joan's parents lived in California and couldn't come, but three cousins and an uncle eventually turned up. She hadn't seen them in years. Dave's parents were dead and his brother was away on business, but his sister-in-law arrived promptly at 8.00 p.m. and brought along another distant relative. Otherwise, the front door bell never seemed to stop ringing. At least thirty neighbours and friends from Haverville came, along with a dozen people from Philadelphia, and, to Dave's dismay, three of his business partners and their wives. About sixty people poured into the Parnell living room. They included several businessmen, lawyers and doctors, three writers, a portrait painter and the teenage son of the lady from across the street: John was a 'Jesus Freak' and was fated to play a major part in the events that followed.

After the initial socializing and discussion of the family's immediate problems, Mark asked for volunteers to spend time with Joan, Dave or the children. Alternatively, he asked people to contribute whatever help might be useful.

Different levels of support were set up according to the interest, talent, free time and plain curiosity of members of the group. Joan chose Mark; Ingrid, a neighbour and novelist; Hans, the painter; and Cathy and Toby, other neighbours, to be with her. She rejected the help of any relatives and anyone having anything to do with psychology except Mark. She neither accepted nor rejected John, but he chose her because 'she was so close to God'.

A rota was set up to ensure that someone was with Joan all the time. A second rota dealt with the children, a third the housework. Complementing this, Dave's colleagues agreed to divide up his work in order to allow him to spend more time at home and to allay his intense anxiety about loss of income.

Those who were not directly involved with Joan or Dave supported those who were. Thus, a number of women volunteered to do the shopping for Ingrid and Cathy. This allowed them more time for Joan. It also meant that they did not have to worry about their own domestic problems. Without this secondary support, the primary helpers would have found it much harder, even impossible, to carry on.

That night Joan managed to catch a couple of hours' sleep. It was a respite from all the tension of the previous few days. Then, in the morning, she entered the full fury of her psychosis. First, she attacked Dave with a hammer, screaming that he had hammered her into the ground, and she was going to have her revenge. Then, after a period of restraint, she tore off her clothes, ran out of the house and made a beeline for the woman across the street. Fortunately, she was headed off by John who had also awoken early in order to meditate. He thought she had tuned in to his meditations and invited her to join him. Joan agreed. She went home, draped herself in a blanket and sat hours holding John's hands. Later, as the agitation returned, she started to tremble. In response John hugged and held her for hours more.

By Sunday Joan had not eaten for days, her skin was pale and cold, her fury was unabated. Then, after a torrent of moans and screams she began to tremble so hard that the ground literally shook from under her. John tried to talk with her, but to no avail. Refusing to be rebuffed, he held her as tight as he could and continued to hold her all day.

In the evening everything began to change. Joan opened her eyes and asked for some tea. Her shaking diminished, then stopped. Days later, Joan recalled the events of the Sunday. She had been shaking with fear because she had thought that her very being, body and soul, had been in imminent danger of falling apart. By holding her John had saved her life by keeping her together. Joan also recalled that she had been very angry, so angry that she was certain that the world was about to blow up. By holding her John had prevented the world from exploding. The denouement occurred when she realized that no matter how angry she was, her body was not going to fall apart and the world was not going to be destroyed. Consequently, there was nothing to be afraid about.

The family made a rapid recovery. Joan rediscovered reservoirs of affection for Dave and the boys. Within a short time she resumed the care of the children and the running of the household. The boys were very pleased to have their mother back and stopped wetting their beds. Dave remained depressed but began to feel more optimistic about the future of the family. He tended to come home earlier from work and spend more time with the kids. One thing didn't please him and no sooner did Joan announce that she felt better, than he booted John out of the house. He said he appreciated all his help but that his wife no longer needed to hold hands with anyone but him. John expressed regret that Joan could not continue her meditations; she had such wonderful 'vibrations'. Then he 'split' to join a commune in Texas.

The whole episode lasted six weeks. The crisis peaked over two weeks. At no time was a psychiatrist asked to intervene. At no time were any medicinal drugs prescribed or taken by any member of the Parnell family. The group as a whole tended to rely on tobacco and alcohol for whatever biochemical relief they obtained.

In the four years subsequent to this incident neither Joan, Dave nor the boys have had to receive psychiatric help. Joan has gone through several periods of depression, but nothing equal to what I have just described. She has emerged from her psychosis feeling stronger and much more able to cope with her family and her life. All her friends and relatives agree that she is a changed person, not nearly as shy and withdrawn as she used to be, and much freer with her affection as well as her anger.

Chris and Sam are doing well at school. They had a rough patch with nightmares after Joan recovered but have not shown any troubles since then. Dave is doing well in his business, but still remains a bit irritable when at home. If anything, he has taken over as the tense one in the family.

The kind of intervention which I have described with the Parnell family is known as network intervention or network therapy. It is based on the premise that individual examples of emotional disturbance are rooted in the malfunctioning of a larger family and social system. The malfunctioning may include acts of omission as well as acts of commission. The former refers to an absence of needed interpersonal support. The latter consists of specific attempts to confuse, bind, scapegoat and upset one person by another.

Perhaps the first step that the network therapist must take is to assess the nature of the significant social system of which a person is a member. Obviously, the family, especially the nuclear family – father, mother and children – represents the core of a person's life. At other times, or in cultures other than the West, this family core would be greatly extended to include grandparents, uncles, aunts, cousins, and so on. Nowadays, most people's significant family relations are limited to the nuclear family and a few fragments of the extended family. But this social lacuna is often made up by friends, neighbours, business acquaintances, and so forth. In the case of Joan Parnell, her significant social relationships included many people who were not related to her by blood, but by proximity. If you take Joan as the arbitrary centre of her social network, you can quickly see that her immediate family – husband and children – were not sufficient to cope with her needs for emotional expression. Her nuclear family were away in California and her extended family were dispersed all over the United States and were not of much help. Joan's most important relationships involved her friends and neighbours. But at the beginning of her breakdown these relationships were not sufficiently intense, either spatially, in the number of people, or temporally, in the amount of time they spent with her, to be able to alleviate her distress.

Moreover, if you take the Parnell family as the arbitrary centre of a large social network, you can see that the network was too diffuse and insufficiently organized to be able to prevent the threatened breakdown, not only of Joan, but of the whole family. Therefore, in this case omissions, or the absence of support, exemplify the primary malfunctions of the Parnell social system. Here the essential task of the network therapist was to mobilize the network for close and prolonged contact. Given such intense and intensive support, the family could stay together and Joan could go through her psychosis. Alternatively, Joan might well have remained chronically depressed or suicidal, the boys might have manifested severe behavioural disturbances and the father might have had business difficulties, started to drink heavily or developed some severe physical illness. All these were likely outcomes. The group outcome would have been the breakup of the family.

The American psychiatrist, Dr Ross Speck, has pioneered the field of network intervention. He has demonstrated that there are many occasions where the family is too weak – either in terms of the personalities of its members or in numerical strength – to help one or more of its members when they are distraught.[1] He points out that if the family provides the primary social context for the individual, then the primary social context of the family must be the total relational field of and around all the members of the family, that is, its social network. If the family is too weak to help one of its members (the very weakness of the family may even be producing the damage), then you must turn to the family's social network in order to produce changes between individual members of the family and in the family itself.

Often dramatic results can be obtained where all other treatments have failed. Ross has told me of one such situation involving an inseparable mother–son pair whom he nicknamed the 'Siamese Twins'.[2] The mother, Mrs Stein, was fifty-four years old and had lost her husband many years before. The boy, Saul, was twenty, looked much younger and hardly ever left his mother's side. He had been diagnosed as 'schizophrenic' and had had many different treatments including drugs, individual counselling, electro-shock, and hospitalization. Nothing helped. Doctors had then told his mother that there was only one other hope for her son: lobotomy. Mrs Stein had come to Ross in desperation. She wanted her son to be cured, but didn't think that brain surgery was the answer. Could he do anything?

Ross listened to their life story. He realized that the boy's 'schizophrenia', as manifested by temper tantrums alternating with periods of withdrawal, was a direct reflection of the deeply entangled, soul-destroying relationship each had with the other. He thought for a few moments, then got up, shook his head and said, 'Sorry, there is nothing I can do.'

Both mother and son tried to protest but to no avail. Sadly they made for the door. Just as they were about to exit, Ross exclaimed, 'Hold on, there is one thing we could do. But no, you would never agree, you'd better go.'

The Steins implored Ross for his help. They said they would do anything. Ross replied, 'It seems to me that both of you are like two orphaned children. What you need are some parents. Go down to the street and ask the first two people you see if they will be your parents. Tell them that in exchange, they will get free psychotherapy.'

'That's crazy!' exclaimed the boy, but after much hesitation, he and his mother went to the street and convinced a passing man and woman to return to the office with them. Ross invited the passers-by to join the family as mother and father to Saul and his mother. Some meetings were held. However, the arrangement did not work out. Finally, the mother decided to invite her sister and brother-in-law to act as the surrogate parents.

The Steins' problem was that after Saul's father had died, his mother gradually drifted away from her husband's family as well as her own. Then she surrounded her son with all the interest and energy which she had previously invested in the family. Afterwards, Saul never managed, or was allowed, to form a relationship with anyone other than his mother. During his adolescence this mother–son relationship became suffocating, as he had nowhere else to direct his sexual energies. Moreover, his desire for autonomy went unnoticed. He could only rebel by hyper-aggressive behaviour towards the mother, or withdraw, and allow her to take care of him like an infant. Since he had no one to turn to for outside advice he could not get a perspective on what was happening. Perhaps the only strangers he met were the doctors to whom he had been sent for treatment. They only confused the situation by calling him sick. Moreover, his mother took up their view and redoubled her attempts to 'nurse' him back to health.

Ross explained that the function of the surrogate parents would be to provide support for both mother and son as well as help the mother to direct her interest towards someone other than the son. He arranged weekly meetings with the foursome and held long discussions about the new 'marriage' in addition to the mother and son's 'marriage'. He also questioned them at length about all their relatives and friends.

After some months Ross remarked that the problem was

indeed very difficult and suggested that it might help if the 'family' would agree to convene a meeting of all the friends and relatives about whom they had been talking. He intimated that the 'family' as a whole needed support and that they might find such support amongst their extended social circle.

The four people hesitated. They hadn't seen many of their relatives in years. But they were also fascinated by the idea. So they organized an evening meeting at the home of one of the relatives. Eventually weekly meetings were held over a period of many months. Upwards of three dozen men and women regularly attended. They represented seven families, four of whom were blood relatives of the original mother-and-son couple, and three of whom were friends and acquaintances. The network called itself 'The Family of Families'.

Ross tried to maintain a neutral role at these meetings. He avoided taking sides and focused his comments on the presence or absence of relationships between husbands and wives, brothers and sisters, fathers and sons, and others that seemed helpful or harmful to all concerned. Significantly, old feuds and angers that had been stored up for years exploded upon many a network get-together. Uncle Abe remembered that Aunt Eve hadn't paid him back the fifty dollars he had loaned her twenty-five years previously. Hymie Greenberg recalled that his sister hadn't come to his wedding. And so forth. On one occasion a riot erupted and the neighbours called the police; all this in a group of 'nice', well-off Jewish families, none of whom had ever previously had a brush with the law.

The goal of the network meetings was to 'alter the relationships between individual persons and the families throughout the network in order to change the state of the network as a whole – increasing communication and human relationships, strengthening bonds between people and removing pathological "double blinds" '.[3] With the 'Family of Families' this goal was achieved within a few months. Grudges were resolved, broken relationships were started up again, and the degree of interaction between various members of the group was greatly increased. Mrs Stein became re-involved with relatives and friends and stopped pestering her son so much. Saul, in turn, made the acquaintance of several boys and girls his own age and took a job in a firm owned by an uncle. Moreover, he decided to move into his own flat and refused to give his mother a key to it. Finally, as if to add insult to injury, he found a girlfriend who began living with him. All this with a young man who had been recommended for a lobotomy only one year earlier.

The disturbance in the Stein social circle exemplifies many acts of commission as well as omission. Saul had been thoroughly confused, bound and hounded for years by a mother who herself was very depressed. This depression had been aggravated by a virtual ostracism on the part of her family when Mr Stein had died. Re-establishing her social network not only compensated for the omissions, but it also helped to correct the scapegoating process which both mother and son had had to endure over many years.[4]

The problems of the Steins, the Parnells, and many others whom I have discussed, give rise to the essential question, 'How can people, despite their personal and general conflicts, still live together?' Long ago this very idea excited the attention of Catharine Ginsberg, psychotherapist and founder member of the F A B Y C (Family by Choice) communities, in Richmond, England.[5]

Mrs Ginsberg had originally trained in education and

social work. She left Nazi Germany in 1934 and eventually settled in Israel with her husband and children in search of a new life.

During this period she thought that the kibbutz afforded the means for people of different backgrounds and needs to come together without destroying each other. But she observed that relationships in the kibbutz were cemented together more by a common response to external danger than by a working through of the tensions that continued to divide many of the people who lived in the communities.

In 1947 Catharine came to London and commenced the practice of psychotherapy. She noted that

Even today, in this so-called enlightened age, psychological illness is still generally described by the contemptuous phrase, 'being out of one's mind – "verrueckt" '. What does it really mean if one asks for the original meaning of this German word 'verrueckt'? A chair or table is 'verrueckt' when it is out of its proper place. So it is with psychological illness. Man too is then 'displaced', outwardly and inwardly: he is in a displaced relationship to himself, to others, to the world. The word 'patient' has also been degraded by much use. The 'suffering person' is often no longer seen in his or her true value but made into an object and then 'handled' as such. Even those most ill were suffering human beings who were not made to be 'handled'. Such clarification was essential for me so as not to find myself in the position of becoming a false authority for the ill person. In therapy and in working together the main concern was to help them to find their proper place, both inwardly and outwardly.[6]

Catharine further concluded that the proper place for a person to find himself and be helped emotionally was the family, not the nuclear family which was too small and constraining, but the extended family. This extended family was to be a family by choice, not necessarily comprising blood relations, rather significant relations, friends, companions with whom you could share a life. In this new family group or community, psychotherapy (in addition to individual psychotherapy) would provide a continual process of emotional assessment. The community would serve the individual needs of all its members and would stay together, not by force of external threat or ideological necessity, but by the development of inner awareness and tolerance, both personally and communally.

FABYC was established in 1953. The original group included Catharine and about a dozen patients and ex-patients. By 1975 the community had grown to eighty members, including forty-three adults and thirty-seven children – aged from a few months to twenty-five years.

In the beginning members shared a house. Then they dispersed all over London, a period known as the 'diaspora'. Next they found flats in a single apartment block. Finally, in 1963, the community was able to acquire several adjacent houses near Kew Gardens.[7] Four of the houses have been converted into one large dwelling, with reception areas connecting the different buildings. The garden walls have been pulled down and a large communal space has been created which facilitates movement from one house to the other. An additional house next door was a later purchase and a second group moved into it.

The main dwellings and the new house have been divided into nine separate units. Each unit consists of two or more families or single people. Members of each unit all have their own private space, bedroom, living room, bathroom, but they share a common kitchen. Weekly group meetings are held among the seven units which comprise the older members and the two units comprising the newer ones. The community as a whole meets informally, at parties, feasts, or in the summer, in the garden.

In addition, three large communal rooms have been built. One is for discussions, lectures and music. The second is for receiving guests and for communal meals. The third belongs to the children for common work and play.

Much time and effort goes into caring for the children. Every morning a nursery group meets led by one of the mothers who has been chosen by the others because of her interest and talents as a leader. Meanwhile, the other children all go to local schools. The younger ones come home for lunch, taken communally or individually in their family unit, and return to a play group in the afternoon in which children of all ages participate if they wish.

FABYC members tend to organize their lives according to their personal needs, not some master plan. This is possible because the community is run pragmatically, and because it has a decentralized structure which allows for different daily routines. However, by choice, the mothers share a common midday meal and do the housework collectively. Women without children and the men go out to work during the day. Many different professions are represented. They include psychologists, architects, musicians, composers, painters, university lecturers, an actor, a TV director, a publisher, an engineer, a chemist, a librarian, a personnel manager, a civil servant, a business man, a taxi driver, a social worker, a secretary, a teacher and a potter. The mothers prefer to stay at home during the day and look after the children, but, if they wanted to work, it would certainly be possible for them to do so.

The physical facilities are very comfortable. But the atmosphere belies an intense turmoil that may be going on in and between people. This turmoil may be brought about by a return of old problems or new problems which arise as children grow up and people change. These issues are usually dealt with in the weekly meetings, or in 'mini-groups' where people choose a few others to join a discussion of their problems. Also, everyone is free to consult with the psychotherapists in the community on an individual basis.

There are many examples of these conflicts depicted throughout the buildings. Catharine encouraged people to paint and the walls hold many paintings and drawings concerned with despair, guilt, hate, murder, sex, and so on. Obviously, there is a great deal of emphasis put on creative work in F A B Y C. The healing potential of such work is attested to by one member of the group, a composer, who, in his youth, was given a lobotomy after a nervous breakdown. Afterwards, he never thought he would be able to compose again or repair the destruction wrought on his emotional life by the operation. Catharine helped him to regain his skills and to overcome his depression by encouraging him to write music for the children. Now his songs continue to be sung in the community, and he is teaching at a training college.

In F A B Y C both adults and children seem to have developed a unique understanding, compassion and forbearance for concerns with which the 'average person' would have great difficulty in coping. These include physical illness, adolescent rebellion, separation – as the children grow older and leave home – and especially death. Catharine died in 1973. She was the great mother, the moving spirit, the prime link between everyone in the group. Some members doubted whether the community could continue. Catharine thought that it would and encouraged people to talk about the possibility of her death long before it happened. And, since 1973, F A B Y C has continued to prosper. There is no longer one central leader to whom everyone turns. The work is divided according to individual talents and personal presence. There is one therapist to whom people turn most for emotional support and another person provides the administrative skills and keeps the books. Moreover, many important tasks are routinely accomplished by others, who also prefer not to be mentioned by name. The brevity of my descriptions does all of them an injustice. Several books could hardly begin to touch upon the richness and complexity of the F A B Y C community.[8]

F A B Y C represents the logical continuation of several major strands of personal and interpersonal support which have been percolating through the psychiatric profession over the past one hundred years. Amongst these is milieu therapy – the use of a structured environment to assist people who have been diagnosed 'psychopathic'. The effectiveness of this work has been demonstrated by Dr Maxwell Jones and his colleagues.[9] Of equal importance are the group therapies and their sequelae including family therapy and network intervention.[10]

The purpose of each of these projects is to begin by getting people together so that they can talk among themselves and to end by these same people overcoming their social isolation, finding a way to live with themselves and contributing to a collective effort for the benefit of everyone concerned.

Notes

1. Ross V. Speck, 'The politics and psychotherapy of mini and micro groups' (paper presented at the Dialectics of Liberation, International Congress, July 1967).

2. Also briefly discussed in Ross V. Speck, 'Psychotherapy of the social network of a schizophrenic family', *Family Process*, 6, no. 2 (September 1967), pp. 208–14.

3. Ross V. Speck, 'Psychotherapy of family social networks' (paper presented at a Family Therapy Symposium, Medical College of Virginia, Richmond, Virginia, 19 May 1967), p. 2.

4. Ross Speck and his colleague, Carolyn Attneave, have written an extended discussion of the theory and practice of network therapy which I highly recommend: *Family Networks: A Way toward Retribalization and Healing in Family Circles* (New York, Pantheon Books, 1973).

5. Catharine Kuster-Ginsberg, 'Family by Choice: A "Grossfamilie"' (a talk delivered to the 'Offentliches Forum mit der Evangelischen Studentengemeinde', 10 November 1970, Düsseldorf, Germany), p. 18.

6. ibid., p. 5.

7. F A B Y C is a registered housing association under English law and, as such, was able to purchase the houses in its name.

8. In 1971 a one-hour film was made about F A B Y C and shown on Thames Television. The director was Udi Eichler who is also a F A B Y C member.

9. Maxwell Jones, *Social Psychiatry: A Study of Therapeutic Communities* (London, Tavistock Publications, 1952); Robert Rapoport, *Community as Doctor: New Perspectives on a Therapeutic Community* (London, Tavistock Publications, 1960).

10. Jerome Liss, *Free to Feel: Finding Your Way Through the New Therapies* (London, Wildwood House, 1974).

9 The End of Isolation

It is no surprise that psychiatric treatments may serve to maintain ignorance, perpetuate fear and promulgate violence. These activities simply reflect the predominant ways in our society that adults treat children, children treat adults and adults and children treat each other. If this is not self-evident, it is because we all have a tendency to gloss over the hatred and cruelty directed both to infants and adults when they challenge social taboos and refuse to act as repositories for others' denied thoughts, wishes or emotions. Therefore, one purpose of this book is to demonstrate the 'battered people syndrome', or what often happens in the guise of psychological care and attention.[1] The other is to consider alternative strategies for confronting the tortured realities of men, women and children who might otherwise be so treated.

The basic requirements of such a strategy are that it is non-coercive, validating and integrative. By non-coercive I mean that whatever is done for or on behalf of another person should be non-punitive and should only be done with that person's consent and approval. By validating I mean that those who provide support should remain calm in the face of others' anxieties and should not rebuke their thoughts, feelings or actions on the grounds that they are wrong, bad, immoral, sick, bizarre or alien. By integrative I mean that the goal of the intervention should be perception, apperception, comprehension and unification – as opposed to denial and splitting.

The first step in this direction was taken by Sigmund Freud and his colleagues. They developed the psychoanalytic method and were accordingly able to demonstrate the pervasiveness and significance of unconscious thoughts and thought processes as fundamental determinants of human experience and behaviour. The analytic relationship still remains a predominant yoga or discipline by which a person can confront the sources of his despair and aggression and come to terms with previously denied emotions and aspirations.

Subsequently there have arisen many variations of psychological intervention, both on a person-to-person and a group basis, which are non-coercive, validating and integrative. All use relationships to heal the emotional, physical and perceptual wounds caused by relationships. The ones I have described in this book offer both practical support – an asylum from outside pressures, a surrogate ego – and interpretative help – to accommodate and not annihilate the psyche. They are particularly appropriate in situations of sudden and massive psycho-social crisis, where in response to such a crisis a person has entered an altered state of experiencing reality – psychosis – or where the disturbance obviously involves a wide social field (couples, families, networks).

A primary difference between those who receive interpersonal support and those who succumb to organic treatments is one of attitude.[2] Regardless of how anxious, depressed or psychotic they may be, the former individuals have an interest in and some knowledge of their psyches. They also wish to retain responsibility for their bodies, minds and external relationships. Those who succumb may have an interest in their psychic lives, but no access to or knowledge of alternative treatments, or they may just be overwhelmed by their own distress and others' anxieties about it.

In the Arbours communities we have had a wide mixture of people. Often they come of their own accord, but if not, they must decide on their own accord to stay with us. Only then can their involvement with the network be of benefit to them.[3] When residents remain ambivalent about what they should do, we refrain from making a decision for them. Instead we continue to point out what we do offer – relationships – and what we do not – prolonged physical restraints on their freedom. Frequently a person who does decide to leave will do so by introducing an unusually intrusive, possessive or otherwise overbearing relative – the embodiment of a severe super-ego – to help him tip the balance in favour of other treatments.

Those who have stayed and benefited most have not always been the best educated or most intelligent. Intelligence helps, but it can also be used to perpetuate problems as well as to create a façade of insight in a situation where a person remains emotionally ignorant. What matters is expressive potential, not prior verbal ability. It is better that they are people who are sensitive to or capable of becoming sensitive to relationships – the needs, the nuances, the realities of such. Then they are able to use the human resources of the network in order to overcome their emotional starvation, to dissipate destructive social games and to find, as in F A B Y C, further meaning to their lives.

However, these benefits must necessarily be limited by the fact that they accrue within cultures which themselves are preoccupied with seemingly endless spirals of recrimination and violence. The issue is how to extend individual strategies of psycho-social development in order to affect the larger social matrix. Reciprocally, there is a need to evolve social structures which, for their individual members, are life-enhancing rather than soul-destroying.

Unfortunately, we are still at an early stage in our understanding of social processes. Even the crucial interface between generations tends to be a neglected subject, the province of the novelist rather than the social scientist.

The psychohistorian, Lloyd de Mause, contends that 'the central force for change in history is neither technology nor economics, but the "psychogenic" changes in personality occurring because of successive generations of parent–child interactions'.[4]

In a previous paper I pointed out that the context for the state of interpersonal disturbance called 'schizophrenia' is a large social network extending over several generations.[5] Each generation influences and is relevant to the experience and behaviour of whoever becomes labelled as 'schizophrenic' as well as every other member of the family.

Recently the psychohistorian, Bruce Mazlish, has detailed the many divergent levels of intergenerational pressure and conflict in a study of James and John Stuart Mill.[6] Interestingly, the son, John Mill, suffered a psychological breakdown in his late teens, recovered from it, and went on to surpass his father as a philosopher and political theorist. Mazlish argues that he has:

advanced broad theses about the nature of father–son conflict, the Oedipus complex and generational change in the nineteenth century, about dependence-independence, liberty-authority, masculine-feminine, rational-irrational relations, and a whole host of other such dichotomies or ambivalences ...

Really to understand any one generation, we must accordingly
ascend to the generation before it, and then descend to the
generation after it.[7]

Morton Schatzman has performed a similar service in his
study of Daniel Paul Schreber and his father, Daniel Gottlieb
Schreber.[8] So has Aaron Esterson in his discussion of the
'Danzig' family.[9]

Bruce Mazlish states that the result, a total experience of
the person, has:

enormous social consequences. It is the interplay of the personal and social, of the individual psychic development and the
general political and economic evolution – with each other
'causing' and influencing the other in what I call 'corresponding processes' – that makes for the powerful social change that
we call history.[10]

Concomitantly, the Austrian sociologist, Helmut Schoeck,
has focused on the role of envy as an all-pervasive emotional
force that affects what happens between generations and
amongst people of the same generation.[11]

Envy is a passionate wish to steal or destroy directed
towards possessions and possessors, both animate and in-
animate. Schoeck demonstrates that envy, fear of being envied, and guilt about arousing envy are irreducible elements
of social behaviour. Most people are aware of some of their
envy and act upon it, but don't talk about it. However, they
will try to contain or attack others who manifest envy to an
excessive degree, or provoke it. These have included
'witches', the 'mentally ill' and the 'nouveau riche'.

Interestingly, at the present time when envy and fear of
envy have become institutionalized in our social structure
in many ways there has been an increasing tendency in the
social sciences and moral philosophy to avoid it as an object

of study.[12] Yet envy and its companion emotions, greed and jealousy, are facts of intrapsychic and interpersonal life. In addition to comprising an essential part of the dynamic structure of these two spheres of activity, envy, greed and jealousy provide the impetus for much of the continuing interplay between the inner world of the individual and external social events. It is likely that these emotional forces are as fundamental to social reality as electrons, protons and neutrons are to physical reality.

In order to overcome projected illusions and to creatively reconstitute our relationships with each other it is necessary to see how feelings such as envy operate across generations, and in and between individuals and groups. In other words, the task on the macro-social scale is not dissimilar from that confronting the psychoanalyst on a micro-social scale or the physicist on a sub-atomic scale.

It is possible to conceive of a society where basic human needs and emotions are acknowledged and met rather than repressed or attributed to others. Although for many people such a society is a ludicrous impossibility, there seems to exist at least one culture which has attained a level of interpersonal sophistication which is comparable with Western expertise in science and technology. I refer to the Senoi, an isolated tribe who live in the rain forest of the Malay peninsula. They do not suffer from war, crime or class conflict. Nor do they have the problem of defining 'mental illness' because in the Senoi culture there are few manifestations of what we would consider emotional disturbance or psychosomatic illness.

The Senoi have achieved a high degree of internal and interpersonal integration on the basis of the communal analysis of dreams. This is a method of psycho-social exploration which they pioneered and developed.

The interpretation of and appropriate response to dreams comprises a large aspect of the education of the Senoi child and is an essential part of the intellectual equipment and social skills of the Senoi adult. Every morning, in each Senoi house, the father and older brothers listen to and discuss the dreams of all the children. Afterwards the adults and older children get together and consider their dreams.

Kilton Stewart, the anthropologist who has made an intensive study of the Senoi, states:

The Senoi believes that any human being, with the aid of his fellows, can outface, master and actually utilize all beings and forces in the dream universe. His experience leads him to believe that, if you cooperate with your fellows or oppose them with good will in the daytime, their images will eventually help you in your dreams, and that every person should and can become the supreme ruler and master of his own dream or spiritual universe, and can demand and receive the help and cooperation of all the forces there.[13]

A common dream which arouses anxiety in all cultures is that of falling. When the Senoi child reports a falling dream, the adult answers: 'That is a wonderful dream, one of the best dreams that a man can have. Where did you fall to, and what did you discover?'

When, as often happens, the child declares that his dream did not seem so wonderful, that it had frightened him, and that he had awoken before he had fallen anywhere, the adult replies:

That was a mistake, everything you do in a dream has a purpose, beyond your understanding while you are asleep. You must relax and enjoy yourself when you fall in a dream. Falling is the quickest way to get in contact with the powers of the spirit world, the powers laid open to you through your dreams. Soon, when you have a falling dream, you will remember what

I am saying, and as you do, you will feel that you are travelling to the sources of the power which has caused you to fall.

The falling spirits love you. They are attracting you to their land, and you have but to rest and relax and remain asleep in order to come to grips with them. When you meet them, you may be frightened of their terrific power, but go on. When you think you are dying in a dream, you are only receiving the powers of the other world, your own spiritual power which has been turned against you, and which now wishes to become one with you if you will accept it.

Similar interpretative suggestions are made about other kinds of frightening dreams. After a while the child learns that the forces, images or situations that he fears in his dreams are not harmful but are a source of pleasure, inspiration and self-esteem. Therefore, he doesn't have to be ashamed of or hide the contents of his dreams from relatives, friends or himself, no matter how violent or incestuous they may be. On the contrary, the dreams provide continual opportunities for social action and recognition.

If, for example, a boy dreams that a tiger attacked another boy, he will be advised to tell the intended victim about the attack, to describe how, when and where it happened, in as detailed a manner as possible, and to himself attack and kill the tiger should the dream recur. In turn, the parents of the attacked boy will ask their son to give the dreamer a present and consider him a special friend.

In the case of sexual dreams, the dreamer will always endeavour to awake with a poem, a song, dance or other useful knowledge which will reveal the beauty of his dream lover to the community. Then, the Senoi believe, the dreamer will never have to worry about expressing or receiving too much love in his dreams – nor presumably have to worry about the envy or jealousy of other members of the group.[14]

The accomplishments of the Senoi and other cultures indicate that man does not have to mistrust his impulses and that social relationships are not inherently frustrating or destructive.[15]

While it will not suffice to emulate the Senoi, although they can certainly teach us about dream expression and interpretation, or engage in utopian schemes as a mass denial of envy, greed and jealousy, there are small practical steps which can be taken to diminish the fear and hatred that exist between different peoples.

Thus, it is perfectly feasible to promote a policy of social education concerned with the systematic study of cross-cultural experience. This term 'cross-cultural' does not just refer to national, racial or religious differences. The word also takes into account divergent clans, classes and sub-cultures as well as the temporal gap between generations. It is likely that all or part of the psychological make-up of members of one group may not be continuous with that of another. Rather, these determinants of character may be radically discontinuous. They may be distinct logical types, not comprehensible on the basis of projected assumptions by one person about another who is not a member of the same clan, class, generation, nationality, and so forth.

Empathy is the natural, but capricious skill that makes this project possible, and which also would be enhanced by it. Empathy is the capacity to put oneself in another's place and correctly assess what he is thinking, feeling or intending. It is an essential aspect of establishing relationships that do not become overlaid with misunderstanding and hostility. Lloyd de Mause cites the importance of empathy in the exchange between parent and child. He refers to it as the 'empathic reaction', the adult's ability to regress to the level of a child and at the same time be separate from him. De

Mause associates this empathic reaction with what psycho-analysts call 'free floating attention' or 'listening with the third ear'.[16] For him it is the primary means by which the negative influence of projection (a putting into and seeing of 'bad' or 'alien' parts in others) can be countered. Of course, this holds true for all manner of relationships, not only be-tween parents and children.

At present individuals are taught how to translate words and phrases from one language to another. However, these translations rarely convey a grasp of the intrinsic experien-ces such as conceptions of time and space, memories, bodily sensations, wishes and expectations which lie behind the words. How many Englishmen really comprehend the ex-perience of being French, Americans of being Russian, and vice versa? For this knowledge there is a need to develop a separate discipline incorporating both phenomenology and linguistics. The purpose of such a synthesis would be to create a verbal basis for the rapid communication of the inner sense of differing styles of being in oneself and in relation to others.

Whether in this manner, or others, the problem remains how to develop forms of social organization and activity that are validating, non-coercive and integrative. My hope is that by a multiplicity of effort people can respond to the challenge of life in lieu of the dance of death.

Notes

1. The counterpart of the 'battered people syndrome' is the battered baby' or 'battered baby syndrome'. Many people have observed that the abuse of children is widespread and it is likely that parents kill, cripple or mentally maim more children each year than do cars or any specific disease. This battering of children is not a recent phenomenon. Lloyd de Mause, a

psychohistorian who has made a systematic study of child abuse, states, 'The history of childhood is a nightmare from which we have only recently begun to awaken. The farther back in history one goes, the lower the level of child care, and the more children are likely to be killed, abandoned, terrorized and sexually abused.' (Lloyd de Mause, 'The evolution of childhood', *The History of Childhood*, ed. Lloyd de Mause (New York, The Psychohistory Press, 1974), p. 1.)

The situation of children is very similar to that of people who have been identified as 'mentally ill'. Both groups have been subjected to the massive projections of others. Both have been expected to carry out roles which they cannot, or do not want to play. And both tend to be stripped of responsibility for some areas of their lives and denied it in others. They are forced to remain in an exaggerated state of dependency and powerlessness in order not to grow up or become free. This prevents them from engaging in those very acts – as did the mythical Frankenstein, or the actual Thomas R. – which would most frighten their creators, their companions and themselves.

Significantly, both children and the 'mentally ill' have been subjected to similar forms of abuse and punishment. These include labelling, ostracism, restraint and extremes of external and internal assault as briefly described in Appendix B.

2. In this regard it is important to note the many organizations, state and private, which have sprung up since the 1960s and which have been concerned with community care and self-help. Groups like the Mental Patient unions have striven to give current and former mental patients a new definition of themselves and to prevent, as they say, 'psychiatric atrocities'.

3. The same is true in the case of psychotherapy or psychoanalysis. People cannot be coerced into attaining insight about or achieving responsibility for their thoughts or actions.

4. Lloyd de Mause calls this viewpoint 'the psychogenic theory of history'. (*The History of Childhood*, p. 3.)

5. Joseph Berke and Leon Redler, 'On the multigenerational study of the family', *Arbours Network*, no. 6 (1974).

6. Bruce Mazlish, *James and John Stuart Mill: Father and*

Son in the Nineteenth Century (London, Hutchinson, 1975).

7. ibid., p. 434.

8. Morton Schatzman, *Soul Murder: Persecution in the Family* (New York, Random House, 1973). Daniel Paul Schreber was an eminent German judge whose psychosis, at the age of forty-two, provided evidence to Freud for his theory of paranoia. His father, Daniel Gottlieb Schreber, was a leading nineteenth-century German physician and pedagogue whose writing on child-rearing influenced many generations of German parents.

9. Aaron Esterson, *The Leaves of Spring: A Study in the Dialectics of Madness* (London, Tavistock Publications, 1970).

10. Mazlish, *James and John Stuart Mill*, p. 8.

11. Helmut Schoeck, *Envy: A Theory of Social Behaviour*, trans. Michael Glenny and Betty Ross (New York, Harcourt Brace Jovanovich, 1966).

12. Progressive income tax, confiscatory death duties and the obsessive placating of third-world countries are commonly cited examples of institutionalized envy.

The tendency to avoid envy as an object of study is an example of collective repression – a group collusive effort to eliminate unwanted ideas or memories from a collective familial or cultural consciousness. Helmut Schoeck points out: 'The indexes of relevant periodicals in the English language during the recent years have been remarkably unproductive for the study of the concept of envy. There is not a single instance of "envy", "jealousy" or "resentment" in the subject indexes of the following periodicals: *American Sociological Review*, Vols. 1–20 (1936–1960); *American Journal of Sociology*, 1895–1947; *Rural Sociology*, Vols. 1–20 (1936–1955); *The British Journal of Sociology*, 1949–1959; *American Anthropologist and the Memoirs of the American Anthropological Association*, 1949–1958; *Southwestern Journal of Anthropology*, Vols. 1–20 (1945–1964)' (ibid., p. 8).

13. Discussed by Kilton Stewart, 'Dream theory in Malaya', *Fire*, no. 1 (1967), pp. 4–8; also *Altered States of Consciousness*, ed. Charles Tart (New York, Anchor Books, 1972).

14. Kilton Stewart also points out that the Senoi are masters of using dreams to achieve creative solutions to social problems. In this manner the Senoi have been able to enhance the ceremonial status of women and to break down major social barriers between themselves and surrounding Chinese and Mohammedan populations. ('Dream theory in Malaya', p. 169.)

15. Erich Fromm has listed a number of cultures which he terms 'Life-affirmative' and where there is a minimum of hostility, violence and cruelty. *The Anatomy of Human Destructiveness* (New York, Holt, Rinehart and Winston, 1973), p. 168.

Accounts of other groups which have developed sophisticated and non-destructive social institutions occasionally surface in the press. One such people not mentioned by Fromm are the Muria with a population of 200,000 living south of New Delhi. They have been described by G. Troeller and C. Deffrage in an article in the German magazine *Stern* (August 1972) and were previously discussed by the English theologian Verrier Elwin in his book *Kingdom of the Young*.

16. Lloyd de Mause, *The History of Childhood*, p. 7.

Appendix A: Arbours Crisis Centre

January 1973–February 1977

A. Number of interventions involving a stay or intensive meetings at Crisis Centre 99*

B. Total people involved 153
   Male 80
   Female 73

C. *Age*

0–14 years 12	40–49 years 17
15–19 years 13	50–59 years 11
20–29 years 60	60– years 13
30–39 years 27	

D. *Marital Status*

Married 71	Divorced 8
Single 75	

E. *Nationality*

Great Britain 93	Rhodesia 2
USA 31	Australia / New Zealand 4
Europe 17	Argentina 1
S. Africa 5	

F. *Occupations*

Student 21	Printer 2
Housewife 19	Catering 2
Businessman / woman 10	Journalist 3

* Includes 21 repeats at Crisis Centre.

Doctor 3   Artist 9
Nurse 3   Unemployed 13
Teacher 8   Retired 6
Psychologist 2   Social worker 5
Engineer 3   Farmer 2
Factory worker 3   Other 39

G. *Reasons for Interventions*
   Depression 39
   Acute psychosis 8†
   Recurrent psychosis 15‡
   Mania 3
   Anorexia 2
   Anxiety states 13
   Adolescent crisis 8
   Marital crisis 6
   Other family crisis 1
   Drug addiction 1
   Acute alcoholic intoxication with severe depression 1
   Threatened rape 1
   Other anti-social behaviour 1

H. *Outcome*§
   Returned home 106
   Went to other Arbours community 16
   Went to other community 6
   Went on holiday 3
   Went to stay with friends 4
   Went to stay with relatives 5
   Got live-in job 1
   Went to live in newly obtained flat or house 3
   Hospitalization 7
   Returned to remand centre 1

   † 1st episode, no prior history of hospitalization.
   ‡ Recurrent episode, prior history of hospitalization.
   § Includes total people involved in interventions.

Appendix B: A Partial Survey of the Abuse and Punishment of Children and the 'Mentally Ill'

	CHILDREN*	THE MENTALLY ILL†
Modality	Specific Methods	Specific Methods
Labelling	Attributions of 'badness': the 'changeling'	Attribution of 'madness': the 'possessed'
Ostracism	Spontaneous abandonment as giving children to strangers, or abandonment on hillsides and doorsteps or for adoption; institutionalized abandonment with wet nurses, orphanages, and other places for unwanted children	Gaoling or mental hospitalization especially in places far away from the original community
Restraint	Swaddling, use of cloth, leather, metal and other devices to restrict bodily movement and actions	Chains, strait-jackets, cages, padded cells, enforced separation from members of opposite sex

* Many other examples of child abuse and mistreatment are discussed in Lloyd de Mause (ed.), *The History of Childhood* (New York, The Psychohistory Press, 1974).

† Many other examples of abuse and mistreatment are discussed in Richard Hunter and Ida Macalpine (eds.), *Three Hundred Years of Psychiatry, 1535–1860*, Oxford University Press, 1963. Otherwise textbooks and histories of psychiatry provide a wealth of documented material.

External Physical Assault	Beatings Whippings Homosexual and heterosexual rape and prostitution. Cold baths, showers	Beatings Whippings Homosexual and heterosexual rape and prostitution. Cold baths, showers, dunking
Internal Physical Assault Purges	Enemas (getting rid of bad parts) Emetics (induce vomiting) Blood letting	Enemas Emetics Blood letting (as with leeches)
Bio-chemical	Various medicinals used to shut-up children including alcohol, morphine, ritalin, amphetamines, phenothiazines, etc., etc.	Various medicinals to tranquillize and sedate including alcohol, morphine, chloral hydrate, barbiturates, phenothiazines, etc., etc.
Electrical	Electrical shock machines to counter bed wetting, masturbation, etc.	Machines to produce pain (behaviour therapy) and convulsions (E C T)
Surgical	Castration	Lobotomy

Index

Agnews State Hospital, California, 157, 166
Alcoholics Anonymous, 140
alcoholism, 42–3, 98, 140
amenorrhoea, resulting from E C T, 80, 87
amygdalectomy (amygdalotomy), 91, 97, 100–101, 111, 113
Andy, O. J., 96, 111
anterograde amnesia, 79–80
Appleton, W. S., 50
Arbours Association, 9, 13, 14, 107, 116, 117–24, 131–2, 161, 162, 166, 197
Arbours Association Training Programme, 118, 121–2, 132
Arbours Crisis Centre, 9, 14, 118–119, 127, 129, 131, 139–55, 157, 161, 209–10 (Appendix A)
The Arbours Network, 122
Archway community, 162–6, 172
Asylum (documentary film), 172
Attneave, C., 109, 194
aversion therapy, 21

Baker, Earle, 96, 111
Balasubramaniam, V., 97, 111
Barnes, Mary, 85, 127–8, 132, 172
Bateson, Gregory, 128
'battered baby'/'battered baby syndrome', 204–5
'battered people syndrome', 195, 204
Bellak, Leopold, 138
Benjamin Rush Center for

Problems of Living, California, 138
bereavement, 136–7
Berke, Joseph, 32, 85, 132, 172, 205
Berke, Roberta Elzey, 9, 118
Berry, Sally, 9, 15, 17, 134–5, 140, 144, 145, 147–8, 153, 155, 157
Bethlehem Hospital, 18
Bettelheim, Bruno, 130, 132
Bini, Dr, 72
Birch, John, 65
Blair, Patrick, 62–4, 84
bloodletting, 61, 62
Breggin, Peter, 92, 101, 105, 108, 109, 110, 111, 112, 113, 114
Brewer, Colin, 82, 88
British Medical Journal, 106
Broadmoor Institute for the Criminally Insane, 32
Bronx Mental Health Center, crisis intervention unit at, 138

California Bureau of Prisons, 99
California Council on Criminal Justice, 100
California Department of Corrections, 99
Caplan, Gerald, 136–7, 155
Cardiazol, 65
Cartwright, Samuel, 107
cathartics, 42–3
Center for Studies of Schizo-phrenia, Rockville, Maryland, 166

213

Index

cerebral haemorrhage, resulting from E C T, 80; and from psychosurgery, 92–3

Cerletti, Ugo, 66–9, 72, 79, 84, 85

children, abuse and punishment of, 204–5, 211–12; at F A B Y C, 190–91, 192; hyperactive, 24; psychosurgery and, 96–7; psychotic, 130; runaway, 24–5, 139; Senoi, 200–201, 202–3

Chitanondh, H., 97–8, 111

Chlorpromazine (Thorazine or Largactil), 37, 38, 46, 47, 50–51

cingulotomy, 91–2

civil rights, loss of, 30–31

Clark, Ted, 169

communications theory, 121

community crisis service, 136–7

Conolly, John, 43–4, 56

Cooper, R., 92

Court of Protection, 31

Crawford, Hugh, 172

criminal activities, and mental illness, 17–18; psychosurgery used for control of, 98–100, 112

crisis intervention, 136–57, 160–61

Crow, A. J., 92

cryosurgery, 91

'cultural closure', 142

Dabrowski, Kazimierz, 125, 132

'Danny', 146–53

'Danzig' family, 199

'Debbie', 143–4

Delaware Valley Mental Health Foundation, 168–9, 173

Delgado, Dr José, 92, 109

depression, 53–4, 60–61, 131; crisis intervention and, 143, 154; E C T and, 70–73, 82, 87–8; lobotomy and, 94, 101

de Vigili, Diana, 157

Diabasis, San Francisco, 169–70

diagnostic labels, 23–6

Disulfiram, 43

double blind trials, 81

drapetomania, 25, 33, 107

dreams, role in Senoi culture of, 200–202, 207

drugs, addicts, 98; drug therapy, 12, 23, 31, 37–9, 41–4, 139, 157; as adjunct to social intervention 48–56; as chemical restraint, 43, 44–5, 47–8; 'flattened effect' produced by, 46; muscle relaxant, 80; prescribing by doctors and nurses of, 49–51; social and interpersonal costs of, 45–6; as treatment to reduce distress, 41–2

dysaesthesia Aethiopis, 25

East Tremont Crisis Center, 138

E C T (electro-convulsive therapy), 12, 23, 31, 52, 58–88, 95, 106; cardiovascular changes resulting from, 80; cerebral haemorrhage resulting from, 80; death wish and, 72; depression and, 70–73, 82, 87–8; fractures in, 80; guilt and, 73–4; loss of intellectual faculties and, 79–80; memory loss and, 58–60, 61, 71, 73–4, 79–80, 83, 85–6; schizophrenia and, 22–3, 25, 166, 185; spinal injuries and, 80, 86

Eichler, Udi, 194

electricity, eighteenth-century medical use of, 64–5

electrocardiogram (E K G), 81

electrocoagulation, 91

electroencephalogram (E E G), 81

emetics, 42–3

empathy (empathic reaction), 203–204

endocrine system, effect of E C T on, 80

envy, concept of, 199–200, 206

epilepsy (grand mal seizures), 65, 66, 69, 75, 76, 81, 102, 113
Epstein, L. J., 57
'Eric', 164–5
Ervin, Frank, 99, 100, 101–3, 105, 112, 113, 114
Esterson, Aaron, 199, 206

F A B Y C (Family by Choice), Richmond, 188–93, 194, 197
facial assymetry, 92
family, autonomy of child and, 13–17, 46, 77–9, 185–7; 'The Butterfly Man' and, 116–17; depression and the, 70, 71, 72–3; E C T and, 78–9, empathic reaction in, 203–4; Family by Choice, 188–93; intergenerational conflict within, 198–199; lobotomy and, 105; network intervention and, 175–188
'The Family of Families' network, 187–8
family therapy, 169
Family Treatment Unit, Colorado Psychiatric Unit, 138–9
Fine, Harold, 168
Fine, Paula S., 87
Forti, Laura, 9, 157
Franklin, Benjamin, 64
'free clinics', 139, 156
'free floating attention', 204
Freeman, Walter, 90, 93, 94, 95, 98, 107, 108, 109, 110–11, 112, 114
Freud, Sigmund, 196, 206
Friedberg, John, 80, 85, 86, 88
Fromm, Erich, 207

Galen, 61
Gallinek, Alfred, 64, 84
Gillie, Oliver, 88, 172, 174
Ginsberg, Catharine, 188–92, 194
Gostin, Larry, 33, 34, 35

Goveia, Leonard, 161, 172
greed, role of, 200
Gross, Mark, 176, 177–80
guilt, 70; E C T and, 73–4; lobotomy and, 104–5

hallucinations, 39–40, 94, 103; John Perceval's, 126–7; olfactory, 97–8
Hamlon, J. S., 81, 88
Haverville, Philadelphia, 175
Heaton, J. M., 172
Henry, Jules, 25, 33
Honig, Albert, 168, 173
hospitalization, 12, 16, 23, 25, 26, 27–31, 33–5, 51, 52, 131, 137, 141–2, 177–8; compulsory, 28–9; deprivation of liberty by, 26–31; 'informal', 28; institutionalism and, 30; of 'Karen', 36–9; lobotomy and, 95; 'revolving door situation', 51; voluntary, 28
Huxley, Francis, 172
hyperactivity, 70; psychosurgery and, 96–7, 98, 111
hypnosis, 133–4
hypochondiasis, 70
hypothalamotomy, 91

'identity warfare', 142
institutionalism, 30, 31, 170
intellectual faculties, loss of, resulting from E C T, 79–80; and from lobotomy, 93
invalidation, psychiatric, 19, 21–3; by hospitalization, 26–31; and by labelling, 23–6
Irvinites, 126

Jackson, Don, 125, 132
Jaffe, Dennis and Yvonne, 169, 173
Jansen, Elly, 170–71, 174

Index

jealousy, concept of, 200, 206
'John' (the 'Butterfly Man'), 11,
   115–18, 119, 129–30, 137, 144, 153
'John' (West Indian actor), 52–3
Jones, J. Easton, 83
Jones, Maxwell, 193, 194
'Joyce', 13–17, 18, 20
'Julia', 101, 105
Jurko, Marion, 96

'Karen', 36–9, 45, 46
'Kate', 77–9
Kibbutz, Israeli, 189
kinesic modality, 47
Kingsley Hall, 77, 128, 161–2, 166,
   172
Kohon, Gregorio, 9, 123, 133–5
Kolb, Lawrence, 86, 94, 108, 110

labelling, 23–7, 30, 106, 205
Laing, R. D., 32, 107, 128, 132,
   172
Langsley, Donald, 138, 156
Largactil, 37
Law Enforcement Assistance
   Administration, USA, 112
laxatives, 42
Lennard, Henry L., 47, 57
Levy, S., 82, 88
Leyden jar, 65
Lima, Almeida, 90
Lindemann, Erich, 136–7, 155
Lithium, 52
lobotomy, fantasy life of patient
   and, 105; pre-frontal, 31, 90–
   114; 'partial', 93–4; political
   aspects of, 106–7; temporal, 92,
   101–2, 113; transorbital, 90–91,
   108
Long, Governor Earl, 32
LSD, 54

Main, Thomas, 49–50
'Marjorie', 167–8
Mark, Vernon, 99, 100, 101–3, 105,
   112, 113, 114
Massachusetts General Hospital,
   99, 102, 103
'Matt', 122–3
Maudsley, Henry, 44–5, 46
Mause, Lloyd de, 198, 203–5, 207,
   211
Mazlish, Bruce, 198–9, 206
Meier, C. A., 129, 130–31, 132
Mellaril, 45
Mental Health Tribunals, 34
M'Naghten, Daniel, 18
mechanical restraints, 43–4
medication, psychosis and, 157–8
Meduna, 65–6
Melville, Joy, 154, 158
memory loss (retrograde/antero-
   grade amnesia), ECT and, 58–9,
   61, 71, 74, 79 80, 83, 85–6;
   lobotomy and, 93
Menn, Alma, 161, 166, 172
Mental Patient unions, 205
mentally ill, partial survey of the
   abuse and punishement of, 211–
   212
Metrazol, 65
'Michael', 89
Middlesex County Lunatic Asylum,
   43
Mill, James and John Stuart, 198
Millett, Vivien, 9, 118–19
Modicate, 55
Moniz, Egas, 90, 108, 114
Mosher, Loren, 161, 166, 172–3
Muria people, India, 207

Napsbury Hospital, crisis service
   at, 139, 141–2
National Institute of Mental
   Health, USA, 112
nervous breakdown, rejection of
   responsibility and, 19–21
Netter, Frank, 108
network intervention/therapy,
   183–8, 194

Noyes, Arthur, 86, 94–5, 108, 110
Number Nine, New Haven, Connecticut, 169

Oakley, Haya, 164
obesity, resulting from lobotomy, 93
O'Brien, Barbara, 127
obsessions, 70, 94, 117
old people, 46, 137
olfactory hallucinations, 97–8, 111
'Oretha', 95, 110
Orthogenic Institute, Chicago, 130
ostracism, 12, 26, 106, 205
Other Voices (documentary film), 173

para-linguistic modality, 47
paranoia, 70, 103–4, 157, 206
Parker, Natalie, 60–61, 80
'Parnell, Dave and Joan', 175–84, 188
Peel, Sir Robert, 18
Pennsylvania mental hospital, 64
Pentylenetetrazol, 65
Perceval, John Thomas, 125–7, 132, 153
Perry, John Weir, 169–70, 173
'pharmacological lobotomy', 47
Phenothiazines, 45, 46, 47
Philadelphia Association, 165, 172
Phillips, D. G., 92
physical restraint, 23–4, 26–31
Pippard, John, 110
Pliny the Elder, 61
'positive disintegration', 125
projection, 204
psychoanalysis, 121, 146, 196
psychogenic theory of history, 198, 205
psychopaths, 21, 24
psychosis, 23, 103, 124–31, 146, 154, 157–8, 167, 169–70, 196;

network intervention for, 175–185
psychosurgery, 12, 23, 89–114
psychotherapy, 53–4, 92, 95, 121, 146, 167, 185, 189–90, 205

Rapoport, Robert, 194
Rappaport, Maurice, 157
Reagan, Ronald, 100, 106
Redler, Leon, 161, 162, 163–4, 172, 205–6
regression therapy, 73, 84, 124–5, 144
responsibility, the family and, 16–17; mental illness and, 17–21; social rule-breaking and, 21–2
retrograde amnesia, 71, 74, 79–80, 83, 85–6
'revolving door' situation, 51, 171
rhinencephalon, 111
'Richard', 53–4
Richardson, Elliot, 100, 106
Richmond Fellowship, Surrey, 170–71, 174
'Robin', 52–3
Rose, David, 157
Rosenhan, D. L., 25–6, 33
Rotary Machine, 64
Roueché, Berton, 60, 84
Ruitenbeck, H. R., 172, 173
Rush, Benjamin, 64
Ryan, Tom, 9, 15, 17, 140, 147, 153, 155, 157

Sabbadini, Andrea, 9, 157
St Thomas's Hospital, London, 65
Sakel, Manfred, 65, 66
Samaritans, 139, 156–7
San Francisco General Hospital, 138
Sano, K., 111–12
Saunders, William, 9, 162–5, 172

Index

Schatzman, Morton, 9, 32, 33, 118–119, 131, 172, 199, 206
schizoid defence, 24, 32
schizophrenia, 22–3, 25, 37, 166, 185, 198 ; chronic, 30, 35 ; E C T and, 65, 68, 69–70, 82 ; 'flattened affect' as symptom of, 46 ; lobotomy and, 94, 104, 110
Schoeck, Helmut, 199, 206
Schreber, Daniel Gottlieb, 199, 206
Schreber, Daniel Paul, 199, 206
Scott, R. D., 138–9, 141–2, 156
Scoville, William, 93–4
Second International Congress on Psychosurgery (1970), 96, 110, 111
'sedative surgery', 91
sedatives, 43, 44–5, 49–50, 55
self-immobilization, 23
self-reintegration, 125, 127
senile dementia, 46
Senoi tribe, 200–203, 207
sexual development of adolescents, 22
smell problems, 97–8, 111
Smith, David, 156
'snow phenomenon', 50
social rule-breaking, hospitalization and, 26–31 ; labelling and, 24–6, 32 ; lobotomy and, 95–105, 106–7 ; responsibility and, 21–2 ; 'the schizophrenic' and, 22–3
Soteria house communities, USA, 161, 166–8, 172–3
Southcombe, R. H., 82, 88
Soviet Union, dissenters in mental hospitals, 22 ; lobotomy banned in, 104
Speck, Ross V., 93, 109, 184–7, 193, 194
State, invalidation and the, 19–20, 21–2 ; loss of civil rights, 30–31
'Stein, Mrs and Saul' ('Siamese Twins'), 185–8
Stewart, Kilton, 201, 207
stimulants, 53–4, 55–6
strait-jackets, 23, 43
Succinylcholine, 80
suicide, 53–4, 70, 72, 84, 88, 101, 139, 157, 168
Sweet, William, 99–100, 102, 112
'Sylvia', 155
Szasz, Thomas, 31–2, 33, 34, 35, 85, 108, 114

Tardive Dyskinesia, 45
terror, application of, in treatment of mental patients, 62–5, 66, 73
thalamotomy, 96
'Thomas R.', 101–4, 105, 113, 205
Thorazine, 37
'Tony', 133–6, 137
topectomy, 90
tranquillizers, 14, 37–8, 43, 45, 46, 47, 52, 55–6, 69–70, 94–5, 106, 154, 157, 170
transpersonal defence, 24, 32
'Trouble Shooting Clinic', New York, 138
Turner, E., 92, 108

United States, 33, 34–5 ; community projects, 168–71 ; costs of E C T, 85 ; crisis work, 138 ; hospitalization, 25–6, 28–9, 31, 33, 34–5 ; psychosurgery, 90–91, 91–3, 94, 96–7, 98–105, 108–109, 112 ; Soteria house, 98–105, 108–9, 112 ; communities, 161, 166–8

Vanni, Professor, 66
Varah, Chad, 139, 156
Veterans Administration Hospital, La Jolla, California, 85
Vidor, R., 109
violence, 27, 38, 91, 120–21 ;

violence – *cont.*
  lobotomy used to control, 98–
  104, 106, 113
Violence Clinic, Boston City
  Hospital, 99–100, 112
Vosburg, R., 104, 109, 114

Wales, Byron G., 29, 34
Watts, James, 93, 95, 96, 109, 114
Watzlawick, Paul, 125, 132

Wellesley Human Relations
  Service, 136–7
Winnicott, D. W., 125, 132
women, lobotomies performed on,
  95–6, 101

Yocum, Mike, 172
yoga, 134, 196

Zeal, Paul, 172